AN ATLAS OF DENTAL AND ORAL RADIOLOGY

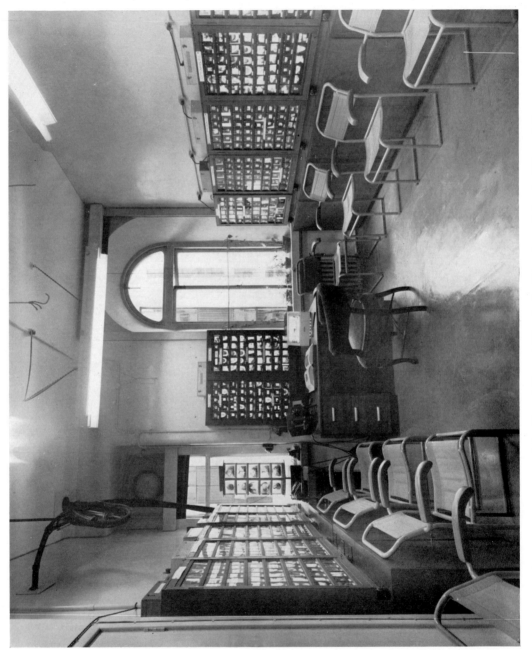

The X-ray museum of the Royal Dental Hospital of London, School of Dental Surgery

AN ATLAS OF
DENTAL AND ORAL RADIOLOGY

BY

SYDNEY BLACKMAN

M.R.C.S., L.R.C.P., D.M.R.E. (Camb.)

Consultant Radiologist, Royal Dental Hospital of London; Director of the Department of Radiology and Lecturer in Dental Radiology, London School of Dental Surgery, University of London; Lecturer in Dental Radiology, British Postgraduate Medical Federation, University of London; Founder President of the British Society of Dental Radiology

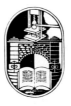

BRISTOL: JOHN WRIGHT & SONS LTD.

1959

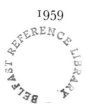

617·60757[1]
BLAC
181061

PRINTED IN GREAT BRITAIN BY JOHN WRIGHT & SONS LTD. AT THE STONEBRIDGE PRESS BRISTOL

TO ALL MY COLLEAGUES
AT
THE ROYAL DENTAL HOSPITAL OF LONDON
AND AT
THE LONDON SCHOOL OF DENTAL SURGERY

Preface

DENTAL practice, perhaps more than any other branch of medicine or surgery, has become closely allied with, if not dependent upon, radiography for diagnosis and control of treatment.

Dental radiography is not as facile as many similar investigations of the body, and there are more radiographic techniques employed in and around the mouth than in any other equivalent confined area of the human body.

The radiographic examination of the teeth is undertaken by placing small films inside the mouth—intra-oral radiography—and by using large films applied to the outside of the face—extra-oral radiography. By introducing films into the mouth in the occlusal or horizontal plane, images of the teeth and surrounding structure are produced in at least two planes and from different angles.

Only the best dental radiographs are capable of a reasonable interpretation, and the techniques available are of inestimable value in the ultimate production of good radiographs.

Interpretation of the shadows seen on a dental X-ray film is the basis of oral radiology and this forms an important and integral part of oral diagnosis. The shadows must be clear, full of detail, and in good contrast. Every radiographic image is a reflection of some part of the tooth formation and its immediate supporting structures.

It is the correlation of the radiographic findings with the clinical examination and the history elucidated from the patient which eventually determines the nature of the underlying condition and the probable diagnosis. Dental radiology demands the practice of perfect standardized radiographic techniques with sound knowledge of the anatomy of the area under examination. Every shadow seen on a film carries its own specific identification and each departure from the normal implies a particular significance.

Any attempt to read a dental radiograph without a good understanding of normal dentition and its many variations in eruption and development is grossly unsound. Any endeavour to identify the existence of disease without profound study of dental pathology is an unwarranted presumption.

This ATLAS OF DENTAL AND ORAL RADIOLOGY is a photographic reproduction from films which, in the main, have been taken during the last twenty-eight years in the X-ray Department of the Royal Dental Hospital, London, of patients seeking routine examination. The author wishes to express his indebtedness and thanks to all his colleagues, past and present, who have been kind enough to render him every support and assistance in the collection and classification of the radiographs and who have allowed him to use their films both from hospital and private practice.

This compilation is divided into three parts and numerous sections covering normal anatomical landmarks, tooth eruption, abnormal development, inflammatory conditions, traumatic involvements, and neoplastic formations. At the beginning of each section an exposition is submitted of the conditions to be presented accompanied by some explanation of the underlying pathology, classification, and sequence of spread and progress.

It is difficult in an atlas of this description arbitrarily to draw a sharp dividing line between true odontological and associated conditions. I have sought the opinions of many colleagues, past students, and practising dental surgeons, and omitted, most reluctantly, examples of dental and facial manifestations of the more rare systemic diseases. It is propounded that dental radiology has become a sufficiently comprehensive study to exclude with justification dental aberrations occurring in diseases which are seen and treated by the specialist physician.

The author hopes that this book will meet increasing needs and demands in dentistry and radiology to provide a reference book for the fundamental interpretation of dental conditions. In addition, it should stimulate a better understanding of dental pathology.

Without the ready and unstinting co-operation of the Photographic Department of the Royal Dental Hospital School of Dental Surgery, this compilation would never have been produced, and I record my unending appreciation and gratitude to Dr. H. Mandiwall, the Director of the Photographic Department, and to his chief technician, Mr. J. Shilland. To my many friends who have undertaken the most onerous task of reading the proofs and checking the illustrations and text, I submit my most profound thanks.

Lastly, I feel that any success that this Atlas may achieve must always be accredited to the Publishers, whose criticisms, suggestions, and general support have made the task a most enjoyable project.

September, 1959   S. B.

Contents

PART I

THE ERUPTION AND DEVELOPMENT OF TEETH

PART II

INFLAMMATORY AND TRAUMATIC LESIONS OF TEETH AND JAWS

PART III

CYSTS AND NEW GROWTHS INVOLVING TEETH, JAWS, AND SOFT TISSUES

PART I

THE ERUPTION AND DEVELOPMENT OF TEETH

SECTION I

Radiographic Appearances of the Normal Anatomical Structures

INTRA-ORAL technique is employed for routine all-round radiographic examination of the teeth and their supporting bone. The small dental film which is placed in the mouth behind the tooth gives an axial view of the tooth from crown to apex. The occlusal film which is introduced in the horizontal plane of the oral cavity presents the position of the teeth as disposed in the upper and lower jaws.

The resultant image of the tooth in its socket must be examined with care and every detail noted.

The crown is observed for its shape, size, and width, the cusps identified and enumerated, the density and continuity of the enamel followed minutely, and the pulp chamber studied for its size, the position of its horns, and contents. In this way, recognition of early caries is made possible.

The root, two-thirds of which is contained in the tooth socket, is inspected for length, shape, and number, and the apex examined for patency and signs of erosion. The existence of hypercementosis is readily apprehended, as is also evidence of resorption of the root.

The elongated dark area of the pulp canal is scrutinized for its translucency, its extent and formation, the continuation into the pulp chamber, and the presence of pulp stones. Obliteration, partial or complete, of the pulp canal must never be ignored.

Radiographically, the socket wall is depicted as the thin white shadow embracing the root of the tooth. It is named the lamina dura, and should be examined for any break in its continuity and followed as it extends over the summits of the bony inter-dental septa. Between the lamina dura and root is a narrow, regular, black area which contains the radiolucent periodontal membrane. This image must be critically scanned for variation in its radiolucency, thickness, and regularity. Normally it is continuous around the whole of the root, widest at the cervical region of the tooth, and thinnest at the middle of the root.

The tooth-bearing areas of the maxilla and mandible are the alveolar processes, and these cancellous bone formations should be surveyed from molar to molar regions, noting their marginal limit in relation to the cervical part of the teeth. The bony interdental septa terminate in a point in the incisor region and gradually become flattened towards the molar region.

The pattern of the bone trabeculation of the jaws and their alveolar processes varies considerably, but there is a closer network formation in the maxilla. Changes from the normal standard are seen as areas of rarefaction, new bone deposition, and recession from the cervical level of the teeth.

The alveolar processes do not appear until the teeth erupt, and with the loss of the teeth, the processes are resorbed, leaving behind the main bodies of the upper and lower jaws.

The two halves of the maxilla enter into the formation of the orbit and nasal fossæ and house the maxillary sinuses. A pathological condition arising from a tooth may encroach upon and displace the normal anatomical structures of the upper jaw. On the other hand, an antral or osseous lesion is often seen extending into the alveolus and involving the teeth and their supporting bone.

The lower jaw completes the oral cavity. It supports the floor of the mouth, into which dental and mandibular lesions may spread. Conversely, morbid changes originating in the salivary glands or tissues of the neck may involve the mandible and the teeth. The identification and position of the palatine foramina in the maxilla, and the mental foramen and inferior dental canal in the mandible, are important factors in radiological interpretation.

To the ever-present bugbears of distortion, the superimposition of extraneous shadows in dental radiography is continually a source of doubtful diagnosis. The overlying of external opaque images upon dental films may emanate from salivary calculi in the submandibular or parotid glands or from calcified cervical or facial lymphatic glands.

Arthroses of the temporomandibular joint have become a subject of interest and concern to the dental surgeon. This demands specialized radiographic visualization of the joint and sound appreciation and realization of the many diseases and abnormalities which affect this structure.

It is therefore obvious how essential it is to acquire a good basic knowledge of the anatomical structure of the maxilla and mandible and of the development and growth of the teeth.

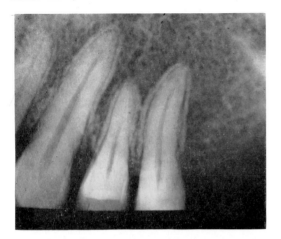

Fig. 1.—Tooth in socket. The crown is capped by a dense white shadow tapering down to the neck of the tooth. The root is peg-shaped. The dark elongated area of the pulp canal situated within the root is surrounded by an opaque homogeneous shadow of undifferentiated dentine and cementum. The shadow of the periodontal membrane is the thin regular dark line between the root and the socket wall.

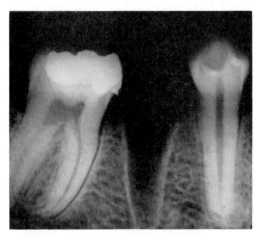

Fig. 2.—Empty socket. The lamina dura is the socket wall and is seen as a linear, white condensed cortical bone bounding the conical socket indentation in the alveolar process. It is not always sharply defined, and the thin buccal and lingual walls of the socket rarely cast any definite shadow across the root. The interdental septa are the projecting cancellous bone supports between the teeth, and their summits should reach the cervical level of the teeth.

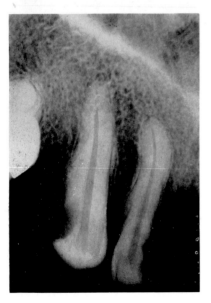

Fig. 3.—Upper central region. The pattern of the bone trabeculation in the upper jaw varies greatly, but usually it is of the close network formation. In the mandible the pattern is more open.

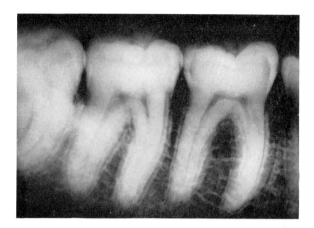

Fig. 4.—Mandibular molar teeth. The molar teeth are multi-rooted with the four cusps of the crown covered by the tapering enamel. The large pulp chamber within the crown receives the pulp canals of the roots. The summits of the bony interdental septa between the molar teeth are flattened and appear to have lost their condensed alveolar margin.

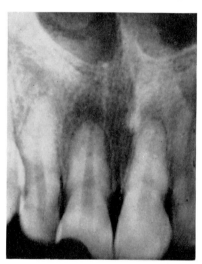

Fig. 5.—Upper incisor region. The crowns of the upper central teeth are wide and the bony interdental septa pointed. The midline suture runs vertically between the central incisors. The radiolucent areas at the upper part of the film are the shadows of the nasal fossæ, separated from each other by the nasal septum which arises from the anterior nasal spine. The shadow of the inferior turbinate bone is shown in the right nasal fossa.

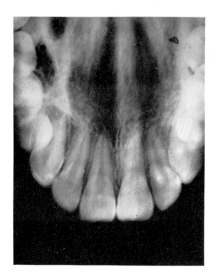

Fig. 6.—Occlusal view of the maxilla. The inter-maxillary suture lies between the two halves of the premaxilla bone. The anterior loculi of the maxillary sinuses may be seen, bilaterally, on the palatal aspect of the premolar teeth. Further back, on either side are the dark circumscribed areas of the orbital entrances to the nasolacrimal canal.

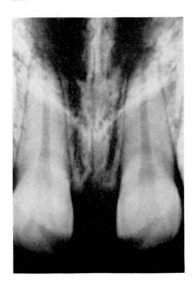

Fig. 7.—Diastema. A median diastema is a non-pathological separation of the upper central incisor teeth. The summit of the intervening bony septa is broadened and flattened. The condition is often caused by a hypertrophied lip band extending from the gingival margin over the alveolar ridge. It may also result from the retention of deciduous or supernumerary teeth.

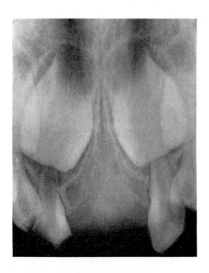

Fig. 8.—Diastema in the first dentition. The upper central deciduous teeth, in a girl aged 5 years, are widely separated. The alveolar margin of the premaxilla is grossly malformed, and the diastema will be continued between the permanent central incisors, which show marked divarication.

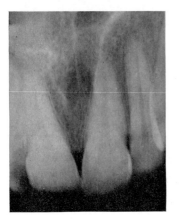

Fig. 9.—Anterior palatine fossa. The well-defined radiolucent dark area between the apices of the upper central teeth in the midline is the image of the anterior palatine fossa. The median suture simulates a fracture of the bony interdental septum.

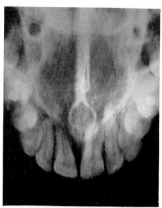

Fig. 10.—The anterior palatine fossa is seen in the occlusal view of the maxilla. The margin of the fossa appears to have a thick cortical bone and is often mistaken for a midline cyst. The radiolucent floors of the nasal fossæ are veiled by the thin plates of the palatal processes roofing the mouth.

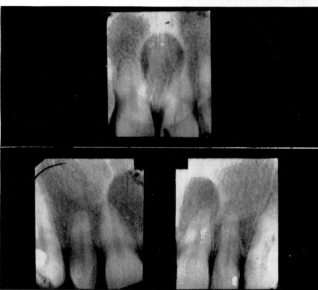

Fig. 11.—Three intra-oral views of a large anterior palatine fossa in the same patient. The shadow of this fossa is shifted by deviation of the X-ray tube to either side of the midline. In all three views the lamina dura and periodontal membrane shadows of the upper central incisors are unimpaired and the apices of the teeth show no signs of disease.

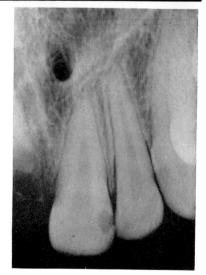

Fig. 12.—An accessory foramen is seen to the left of the median suture. Between the left central and lateral incisor teeth there is an elongated radiolucent shadow of a nutrient artery canal in the bony inter-dental septum.

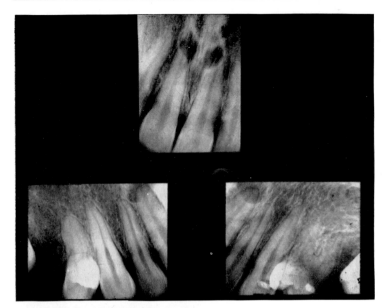

Fig. 13.—The four anterior palatine foramina are seen without an anterior palatine fossa shadow. This condition is more often seen in the lower mammalia.

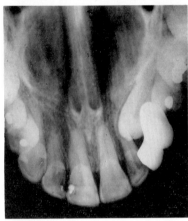

Fig. 14.—Occlusal view of the maxilla showing two separate anterior palatine foramina lying on either side of the midline suture, just beyond the apices of the upper central incisors. There is no image of an anterior palatine fossa.

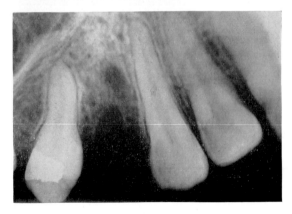

Fig. 15.—Upper premolar region. The first upper premolar tooth has been extracted and the sockets of the two roots are depicted. The history of the recent extraction of the tooth should obviate misinterpreting the shadows as localized residual infection.

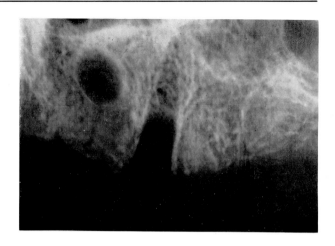

Fig. 16.—Empty socket of 4|, of an outstanding tooth. Liable to be mistaken for an accessory foramen or a cystic condition.

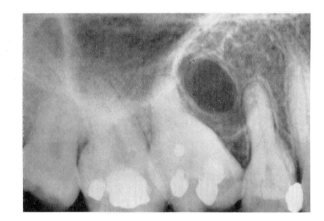

Fig. 17.—Empty socket of 5|. This tooth was also outstanding. In view of its position, the radiolucent area might be confused with the appearance of a residual cyst or a forward loculus of the right antrum.

Fig. 18. — The crescentic white line running across the apical region of 5| and across the distal half of the root of 6| is the shadow of the floor of the antrum. Both upper premolar teeth are double rooted.

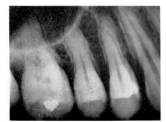 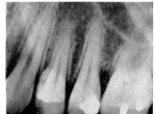

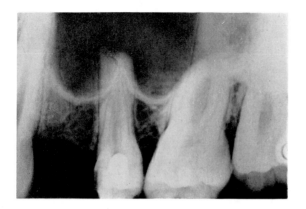

Fig. 19.—This shows the classical radiographic dark **W**-shaped shadow of the antrum dipping down in the premolar region with the illusion of the roots of 5| invaginating themselves into the floor of the antrum.

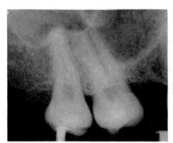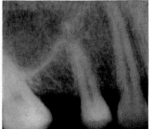

Fig. 20.—The main antral shadow is in 87| region with a forward loculus in the premolar region.

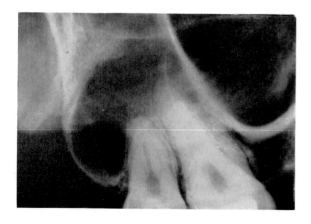

Fig. 21.—The antrum extending backwards is incorporated in the tuberosity of the maxilla. The knowledge of the existence of this anatomical variation is important on account of the potential fracture of the bone in this area if 8| has to be extracted. The crescentic opaque line shadow superimposed upon 6| region is the margin of the malar bone. Last molar tooth has confluent roots.

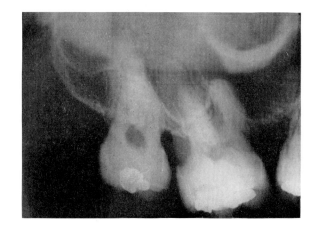

Fig. 22.—Not all of the tuberosity is included in the antral shadow. Crescentic opaque image of the lower part of the malar bone is seen. The apices of <u>87|</u> appear to be invaginated into the floor of the antrum. This is produced by a buccal and downward expansion of the right antrum.

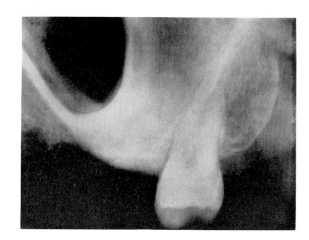

Fig. 23.—The antrum is seen as a radiolucent area through a window-like frame made by the thin wall of the malar bone.

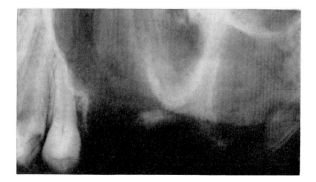

Fig. 24.—The antral shadow is seen extending as far forward as the lateral incisor and canine teeth, and backwards into the tuberosity of the maxilla.

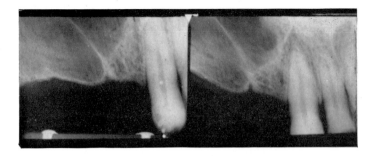

Fig. 25.—The antral shadow in the upper right premolar region is divided into two compartments by a bony septum shown on the film as an oblique thin white opaque line. Often confused as a multiloculated cyst.

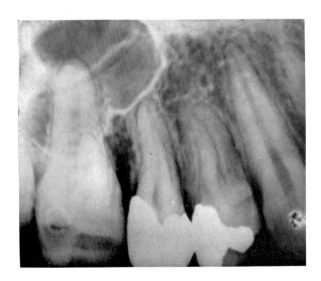

Fig. 26.—An important distinguishing feature in the antral shadow is the presence of channels of nutrient vessels. These are seen as oblique radiolucent lines running across the image of the lower part of the antrum.

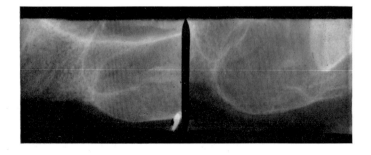

Fig. 27.—The alveolar margin forms the floor of the antrum in the above edentulous area. In the absence of the teeth and alveolar process there is a downward convexity of the antral shadow, and with the presence of the septa the picture simulates a multiloculated dental cyst. The nutrient channels are the key to the identification of the antrum.

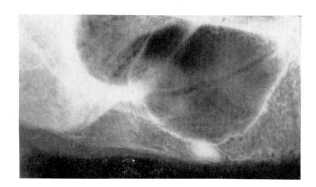

Fig. 28.—The close proximity of a retained root to the radiolucent area is suggestive of a dental cyst in the 654| region. The differentiating features are the non-spherical outline of the antral shadow, the radiating channels, and the absence of continuity between the wall of the antrum and the socket of the root.

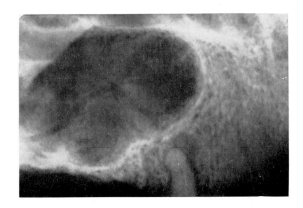

Fig. 29.—There is a chronic apical abscess in association with the retained root in the upper right premolar region. The abscess may penetrate into the antrum and produce an empyema.

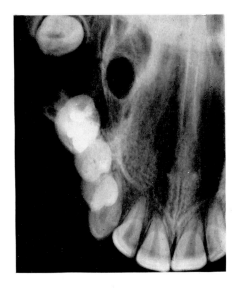

Fig. 30.—The occlusal view shows a large outward buccal expansion of the antrum with the shadow of the orbital entrances to the nasolacrimal canal lying on the palatal side of 7| socket.

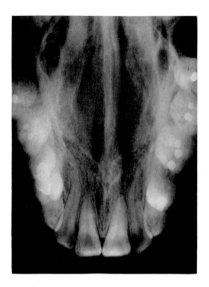

Fig. 31.—The full occlusal view shows the median suture with the radiolucent shadows of the nasal fossæ on either side of it. The two orbital entrances to the nasolacrimal canal are seen symmetrically placed in the molar region. Displacement of the orbital entrance of the nasolacrimal canal is usually a sign of a pathological condition in the molar region.

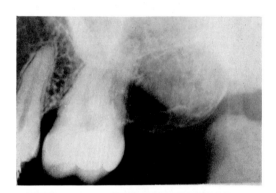

Fig. 32.—Shows the tuberosity of the maxilla with the hamular process immediately posterior to it, and the opaque triangular shadow of the coronoid process of the ascending ramus below the tuberosity.

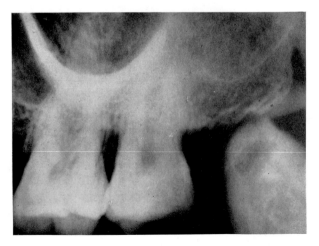

Fig. 33.—The coronoid process of the mandible could be mistaken for a molar tooth. The differentiating points are the absence of a pulp canal, lamina dura, and periodontal membrane shadow.

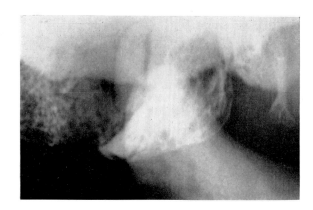

Fig. 34.—The hamular process of the sphenoid bone is shown as a radio-opaque hook-like projection extending downwards and backwards behind the tuberosity of the maxilla.

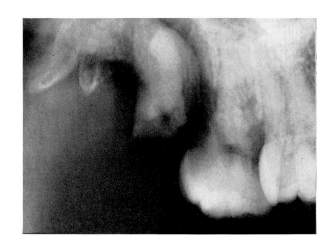

Fig. 35.—Retained roots of 8| lateral to 7|. The exaggerated shadow of the coronoid process is seen overlying the tuberosity of the hamular process.

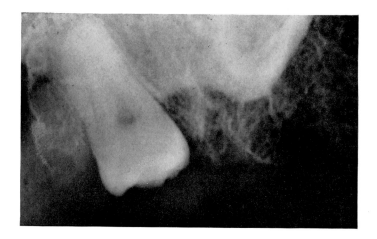

Fig. 36.—8| is unerupted and the opaque shadow mesial to it is that of the lower angle of the malar bone.

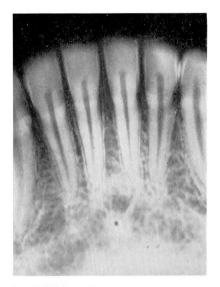

Fig. 37.—The lower four incisor teeth are smaller and their crowns are narrower than those of the upper opposing teeth. The bony interdental septa reach the necks of the teeth and are pointed. The circular opaque area below the apices of the central teeth is that of the genial tubercle with a central lingual foramen. The hazy white oblique lines running downwards and outwards from a point between the apices of the central teeth are the mental ridges.

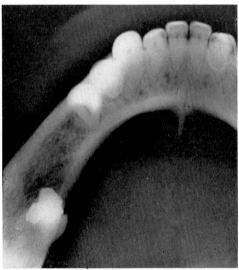

Fig. 38.—An occlusal view of the mandible with the genial tubercle projecting into the floor of the mouth from the lingual aspect of the bone. The black dots seen in the bone around the apices are nutrient foramina.

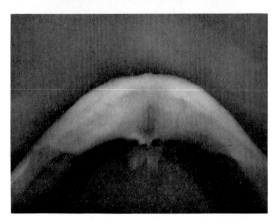

Fig. 39.—The genial tubercles are grossly enlarged almost to the point of exostoses.

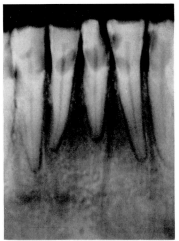

Fig. 40.—The radiolucent lines running vertically downwards between the central and incisor teeth are the shadows of the nutrient channels carrying the incisive branches of the inferior dental arteries.

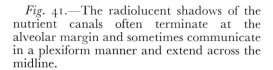

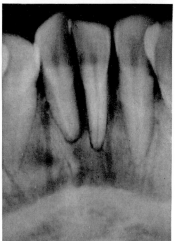

Fig. 41.—The radiolucent shadows of the nutrient canals often terminate at the alveolar margin and sometimes communicate in a plexiform manner and extend across the midline.

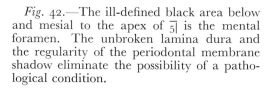

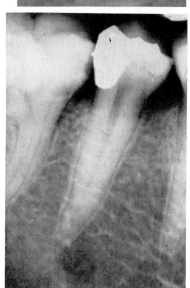

Fig. 42.—The ill-defined black area below and mesial to the apex of ⁵⌋ is the mental foramen. The unbroken lamina dura and the regularity of the periodontal membrane shadow eliminate the possibility of a pathological condition.

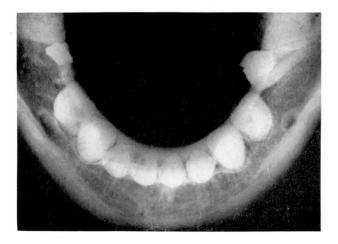

Fig. 43.—Occlusal view of the mandible showing the mental foramina buccal to the premolar teeth.

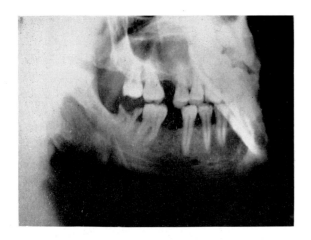

Fig. 44.—The inferior dental canal is depicted as a radiolucent channel running downwards and forwards below the apices of the molar teeth to the mental foramen. The extension anteriorly beyond the mental foramen of the canal is produced by an accessory branch.

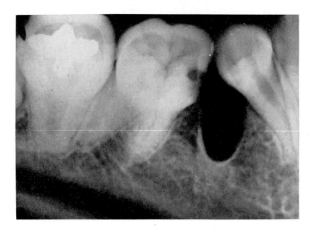

Fig. 45.—The radiolucent area between $\overline{4|}$ and $\overline{6|}$ is the empty socket of an extracted $\overline{5|}$. It has the well-defined cortex of the lamina dura, no connexion with the dental canal, and is open to the alveolar margin.

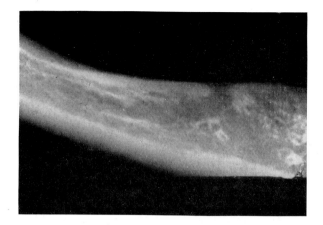

Fig. 46.—Edentulous premolar region, showing the proximal end of the inferior dental canal terminating in the mental foramen which is situated on the free margin of the mandible. There is complete resorption of the alveolar process, and pressure from a denture on the nerve would set up a painful neuritis.

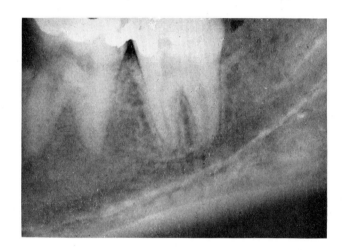

Fig. 47.—Intra-oral view of the molar part of the inferior dental canal. The apices of the 8̄| are in close approximation to the canal shadow.

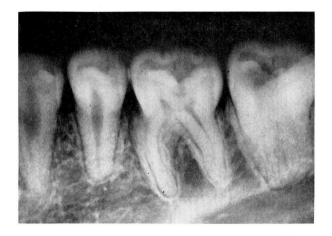

Fig. 48.—The broad oblique shadow running downwards and forwards across the apices of the molar teeth is the mylohyoid ridge. Immediately below this is the radiolucent area of the dental canal.

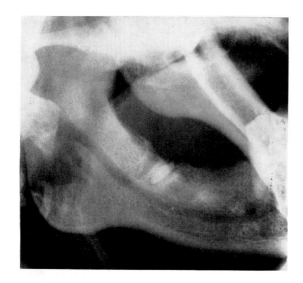

Fig. 49.—A full view of the inferior dental canal from the mandibular foramen to the mental foramen.

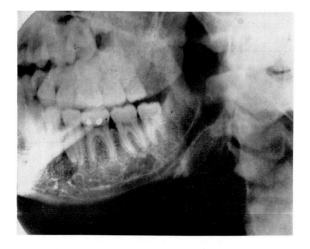

Fig. 50.—The upper end of the inferior dental canal is seen beginning as a funnel-shaped radiolucent shadow, the mandibular foramen.

Fig. 51.—Thinning or apparent absence of network pattern seen below the inferior or dental canal in the molar mandibular area. May be associated with proliferation of hæmopoietic tissue in the red marrow of the bone activated by a systemic demand for blood-corpuscles. The osteolytic changes in the spongiosa may be mistaken for dental cysts or hæmorrhagic cysts.

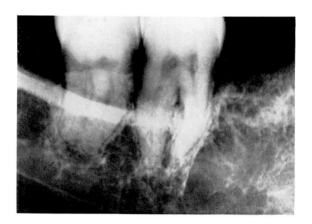

Fig. 52.—The elongated opaque shadow running downwards and forwards over the posterior part of the ramus is the image of the calcified stylohyoid ligament. Pharyngeal space, broad dark elongated area running downwards and backwards across the body of the ascending ramus.

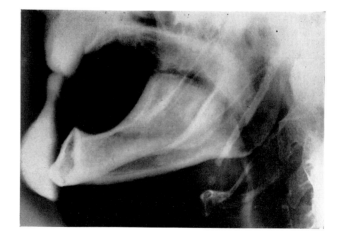

II.—NORMAL TOOTH DEVELOPMENT

1. Intra-oral survey.

2. Extra-oral survey.

3. Bimolar radiography.

4. Topography.

5. Cephalometry.

Normal Tooth Development

THE radiographic visualization of the tooth in the infant depends upon calcium formation in the bony dental crypt. Calcium deposition throws opaque shadows on the X-ray film.

The process of calcification is by no means rigid in its chronology, and many variations in tooth development and tooth eruption are encountered at various levels.

At birth, the mandible consists of two halves connected at the symphysis menti by fibrous tissue. Osseous union is completed towards the end of the first year or at the beginning of the second year.

The inferior border of the mandible is not well developed at birth, and the ramus is mounted at an angle of 150° to the shallow body. The condyles of the mandible are rudimentary, and are still immature at six months of age. The coronoid processes are slightly more advanced and longer than the condylar processes, and the mental foramen is nearer the inferior than the superior border. From six months onwards, with the beginning of the eruption of the teeth, the growth of the lower jaw is most rapid and striking.

The maxilla is composed of two bones, the maxilla proper, and the premaxilla, with the latter bearing the upper incisor teeth. The line of union between these bones is indicated by the premaxillary or incisal suture on the palatine surface of young bones, but rarely persists in adult life.

The maxilla, with its fellow, forms a large part of the face, and besides supporting the upper teeth of its own side, enters into the formation of the orbit, nasal fossa, antrum, and the hard palate. It is composed of a central portion or body, and four processes—frontal, zygomatic, alveolar, and palatine.

The maxillary sinus is an excavated air-space in the body of the maxilla, and is pyramidal in shape. The base of the pyramid is formed by the lateral wall of the nasal cavity with the apex extending into the zygomatic process. The antero-lateral wall corresponds to the facial surface of the maxilla and the postero-lateral wall is formed by the zygomatic surface of the maxilla. The roof is formed by the orbital plate, and the floor reaches into the alveolar process.

There is a considerable variation in size, shape, and position of the maxillary sinus, not only in different persons, but also on the two sides of the same person.

Deciduous Dentition.—The tooth crypt is seen on the radiograph as a sharply defined dark space surrounded by a white, condensed, spherical, thin wall known as the lamina dura. Calcification of the crowns of the deciduous teeth within the crypts takes place half-way in intra-uterine life and is completed at the end of the first year.

When the baby is born, it carries 44 bony crypts in its jaws, the full 20 of the first dentition and 24 of the second dentition. Those of the last two permanent molars on both sides in the maxilla and mandible are not yet formed.

Radiographically, 24 teeth are seen at birth. The crowns of all the deciduous teeth and the tips of the cusps of the first permanent molar teeth exhibit signs of various degrees of calcification.

Permanent Dentition.—All the permanent teeth, with the exception of the third molars, become calcified by the end of the fourth year of life and are clearly visible on a radiograph. Calcification of the third molars may start at about 8 years of age and all the permanent teeth, with the exception of these, should be in their recognized position by the age of 16 years. The permanent dentition with eruption of the third molars should be complete by the age of 25 years.

Calcification and eruption of the third molars show considerable variation. If calcification is not apparent by the twelfth year, it may be assumed that the third molars are absent from the dental arches.

Dental radiography of the child should be carried out as early as possible, but the child's intolerance of a dental film in the mouth makes intra-oral examination impracticable before the fourth or fifth year. On the other hand, occlusal radiography can be undertaken from about 2 years of age, to produce a reasonable view of the upper and lower dental arches.

Extra-oral lateral oblique technique, concentrating upon the deciduous molar regions and beyond, is not difficult in an infant of twelve months. This form of radiographic examination can be extended to the bimolar extra-oral technique. For further information, rotational tomography may be recommended.

Using a craniostat, true lateral radiography is employed by the orthodontist for cephalometric purposes. This can be undertaken when the child is 3 years of age.

By these radiographic methods the existence of the teeth of both dentitions is easily established, and normal and abnormal features of tooth development identified in the first year in the life of the child.

An early radiographic survey will reveal underlying pathological conditions, such as odontomes, which may interfere with normal eruption.

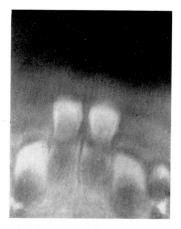

Fig. 53.—Baby, aged 7 weeks. $\overline{1|1}$. Crowns of the deciduous incisor teeth are not yet seen in the mouth, but are well developed in the jaws. The apices of the calcified teeth are wide open. Eruption into the oral cavity begins at six months, with the temporary lower central teeth preceding in eruption those of the corresponding teeth of the upper jaw. (Radiograph enlarged four times.)

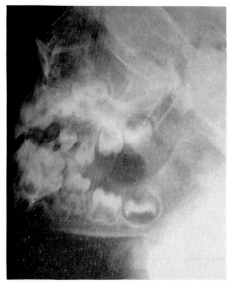

Fig. 54.—Infant, aged 16 months. External oblique view. Calcification of the first dentition is completed in the first year. The second deciduous molar teeth are not fully erupted. The crypt of the unerupted first lower permanent molar tooth, containing a well-formed crown, is lying midway between the alveolar margin and the lower border of the mandible. No sign of the presence of the second permanent molar teeth.

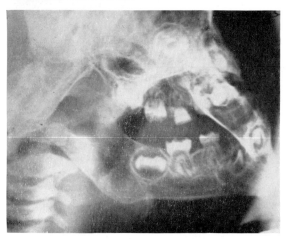

Fig. 55.—Infant, aged 20 months. All the deciduous molar teeth have erupted with advanced root formation. The crypts of the unerupted first lower permanent molar teeth have advanced nearer to the alveolar margin. The ramus of the jaw, with condyle and coronoid processes, is developing well and the mandibular notch and inferior dental canal are seen. No sign of the presence of the second permanent molar teeth.

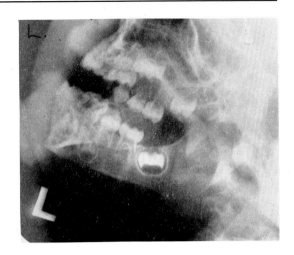

Fig. 56.—Child, aged 2 years. The body of the mandible is elongating and the crypt of the unerupted first lower permanent molar tooth is now anterior to the downward prolongation of the anterior border of the ramus. The eruption of the twenty deciduous teeth is usually completed by the end of the 30th month.

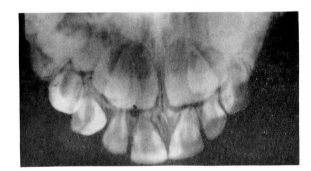

Figs. 57, 58.—Child, aged 3½ years. Occlusal views of the upper and lower jaws, showing the buccal disposition of the deciduous teeth, with the unerupted permanent teeth lying on the palatal and lingual aspects.

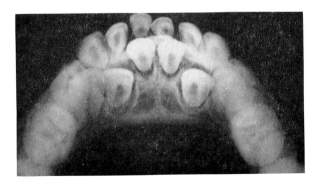

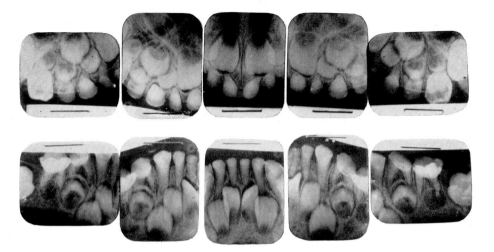

Fig. 59.—Boy, aged $3\frac{1}{2}$ years. The deciduous incisor and canine teeth are single-rooted, with bulbous crowns. Their necks tend to be constricted. The molar teeth are multi-rooted and widely splayed. The crypts of the lower second permanent premolar teeth are seen, but no signs of crown calcification. $\frac{54321|12345}{54321|12345}$. These teeth of the second dentition are seen unerupted with their crowns in advanced stage of calcification.

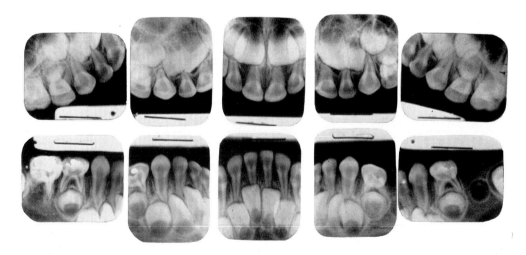

Fig. 60.—Girl, aged 4 years. No signs of resorption of the roots of the teeth of the first dentition. Root resorption begins at the end of the fourth year, beginning usually at the temporary molars and then in the incisors. Early signs of crown calcification of the lower left second permanent bicuspid tooth. The second lower left temporary molar tooth is absent.

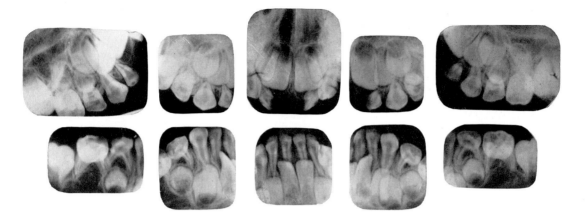

Fig. 61.—Boy, aged 5 years. The upper deciduous central teeth have been shed, and there is active root resorption of $\frac{\text{ed b|b de}}{\text{a|a}}$. $\overline{1|1}$ advancing towards eruption. $\overline{5|5}$, these permanent teeth do not appear to be present. $\frac{6|6}{6|6}$ are at the alveolar margin with the roots partially formed.

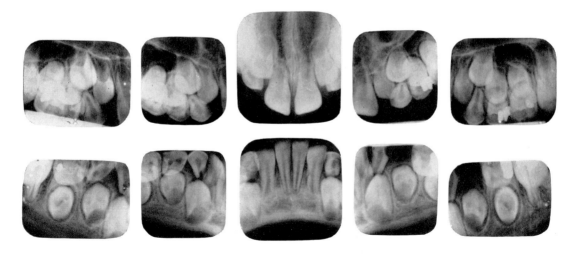

Fig. 62.—Girl, aged 6 years. $\frac{\text{ba|ab}}{\text{ba|ab d}}$ have been shed. $\frac{\text{edc|cde}}{\text{edc|c e}}$ show different degrees of root resorption. $\frac{6 \ 1|1 \ 6}{6 \ 1|1 \ 6}$ are erupted with well-formed root formation. Maxillary canines are far above the dental arch. Mandibular canines are near the lower border of the mandible.

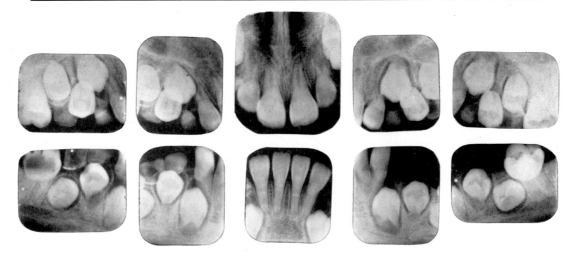

Fig. 63.—Boy, aged 7 years. This is the same child as in *Fig.* 59. $\frac{e\ c\ |\ c\ e}{edc\ |}$ are still retained, but almost completely resorbed. $\frac{6\ \ 21|12\ \ 6}{6\ \ 21|12\ \ 6}$ are fully erupted. Note the phalanx formation of $\frac{543\ |\ 345}{543\ |\ 345}$ with the $\frac{4|4}{4|4}$ at the apex of the triangle. The root canals close within three years of the eruption of the teeth and gradually become narrower. The mandibular teeth erupt and close slightly ahead of those of the maxilla.

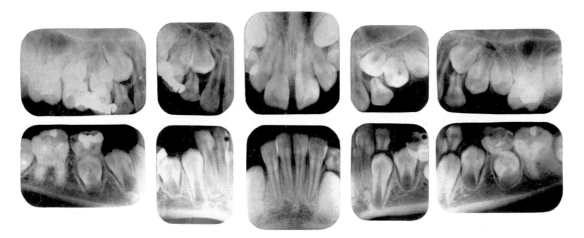

Fig. 64.—Girl, aged 8 years. No other permanent teeth are erupted beyond $\frac{6\ \ 21|12\ \ 6}{6\ \ 21|12\ \ 6}$, although the $\frac{4|4}{4|4}$ are at the very edge of the alveolar margin. The roots of the lower incisor teeth show advanced formation. The calcified crowns of the $\frac{7|7}{7|7}$ are now in evidence.

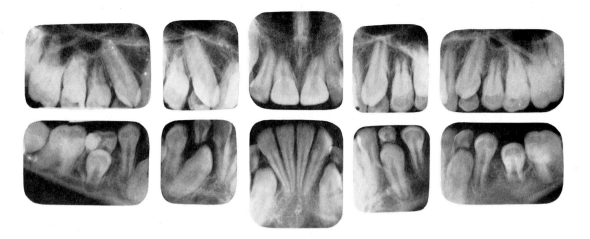

Fig. 65.—Boy, aged 9 years. $\frac{6\ 4\ 21|12\ 4\ 6}{6\ 4\ 21|12\ 4\ 6}$ are fully erupted. $\overline{5|5}$ are at the alveolar margin. $\frac{e\ c\ |\ c\ e}{e\ c\ |\ c}$ almost completely resorbed, but still retained.

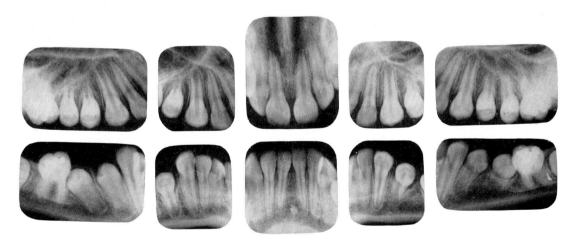

Fig. 66.—Girl, aged 10 years. All temporary teeth are lost during the tenth year. $\underline{654321|123456}$ have erupted. $\overline{7\ 54\ |\ 45\ 7}$ not erupted, but at alveolar margin.

BIMOLAR RADIOGRAPHY

Bimolar radiography is a convenient technique whereby both sides of the face can be depicted upon one film, in the same plane. This method of extra-oral radiography is applicable especially in the visualization of the premolar and molar regions in the young child. The presence, development, and eruption of the permanent molar teeth can be followed and compared year by year, and provide valuable information to the orthodontist.

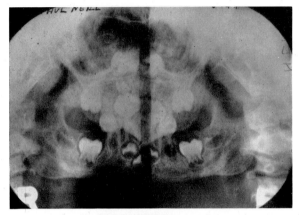

Fig. 67.—Boy, aged 3 years. All the four first permanent molar teeth are shown unerupted, with early root formation. The crowns reveal a high degree of enamel calcification. The cusps of the second permanent molar teeth in the mandible are seen in their crypts.

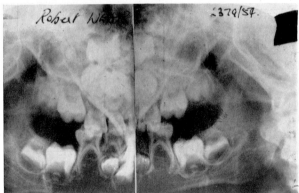

Fig. 68.—Boy, aged 5 years. All the four first permanent molar teeth have reached the alveolar margin. Calcification of the crowns of the unerupted second permanent molars is more advanced. $\overline{5|5}$ are absent.

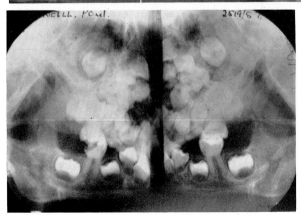

Fig. 69.—Same patient as *Fig.* 67. Boy, aged 6 years. Full eruption of the four first permanent molar teeth which are in occlusion. $\frac{7|7}{7|7}$ calcification of the crowns.

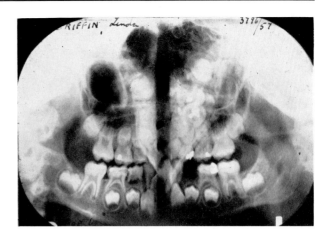

Fig. 70.—Girl, aged 7 years. The molar teeth show no further progress.

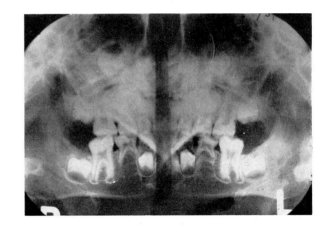

Fig. 71.—Same patient as *Fig.* 68. Boy, aged 8 years. No signs of the presence of $\frac{8\ 5\ |\ 5\ 8}{8\ 5\ |\ 5\ 8}$.

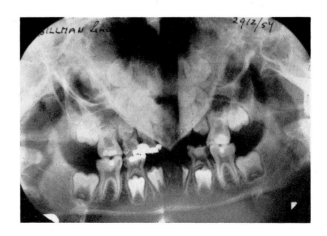

Fig. 72.—Girl, aged 8½ years. $\frac{7|7}{7|7}$ the crowns are at the alveolar margin and the teeth show early root formation.

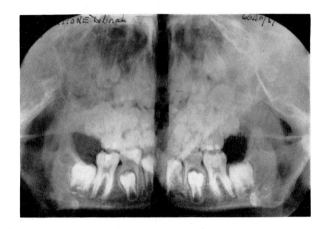

Fig. 73.—Girl, aged 9 years. $\frac{7|7}{7|7}$ appears at the alveolar margin. $\overline{8|}$ first signs of crypt formation.

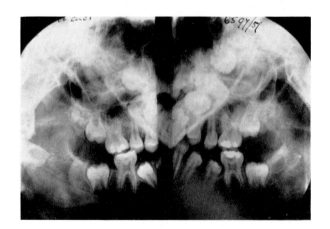

Fig. 74.—Girl, aged 10 years. $\frac{7|7}{7|7}$ the crowns have penetrated the alveolar margin. $\frac{8|8}{8|8}$ radiographic signs of crown calcification. $\overline{8|}$ crypt not seen.

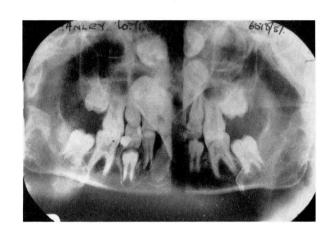

Fig. 75.—Girl, aged 11 years. $\frac{7|7}{7|7}$ eruption proceeding normally. $\frac{8|8}{8|8}$ no signs of crypts.

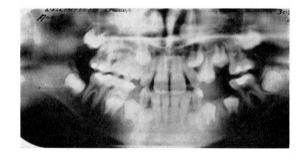

Fig. 76.—Girl, aged 9 years. Rotograph of the teeth. This technique provides a quick survey of the teeth using a single extra-oral film.

CEPHALOMETRY

Lateral skull radiographs are taken with the patient's head held in a fixed position in a cephalostat, the tube being placed at a distance of 6 feet. They are, therefore, very useful not only for diagnosis but also for a serial study before and after treatment.

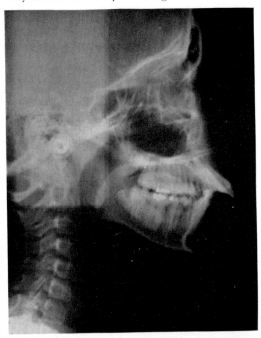

Fig. 77.—Shows a typical case of an Angle's Class II, division 1 malocclusion on a Skeletal II dental base. Note the extreme proclination of the upper incisors and the increased overbite and overjet. There is a postnormal molar relationship.

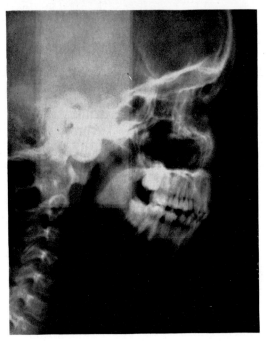

Fig. 78.—Shows an Angle's Class II, division 2 malocclusion on a Skeletal II dental base. Here the upper incisors are retroclined and there is also a postnormal molar relationship.

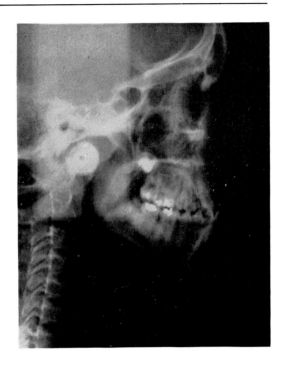

Fig. 79.—Shows Angle's Class III malocclusion on Skeletal III dental bases. Note the short anteroposterior maxillary apical base. (*See also Fig.* 80.)

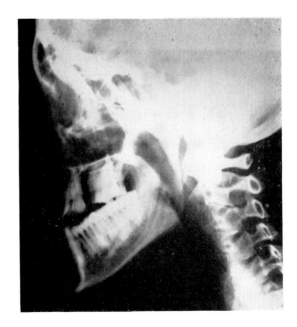

Fig. 80.—This picture, which has not been taken in a cephalostat, shows also an anterior open bite and an increase in the Frankfort mandibular plane angle.

III.—DEVELOPMENTAL ABERRATIONS

1. Premature shedding of deciduous teeth.

2. Delayed eruption of lower central teeth.

3. Maxillary and mandibular canines.

4. Premolar teeth.

5. Transposed and migrating teeth.

6. Submerged teeth.

7. Maleruption and impaction.

8. Anodontia.

9. Supernumerary teeth.

Developmental Aberrations

DEVELOPMENTAL aberrations cover a large and varied field.

Premature shedding of the deciduous teeth is associated with poor general health in the young child. Specific diseases and endocrine and nutritional disorders are often accompanied by early loss of the deciduous teeth. In the majority of the foregoing conditions dental caries and periapical disease are the ultimate factors in the premature exfoliation of the deciduous teeth.

Premature shedding of the deciduous teeth has been reported in cases of systemic conditions, such as eosinophilic granuloma and Schüller-Christian's disease, which affect the skeleton during the period of growth and development.

Delayed eruption, as distinct from impeded eruption, is not a common aberration.

The deciduous teeth are not so frequently affected as the permanent dentition, and in most cases there is a history of endocrine dysfunction.

Individual teeth of the permanent dentition may be retarded or impeded in their eruption. In most cases it may be due to malposition or obstruction, and the tooth may be found to be inverted, transposed, or even migrating from its normal position.

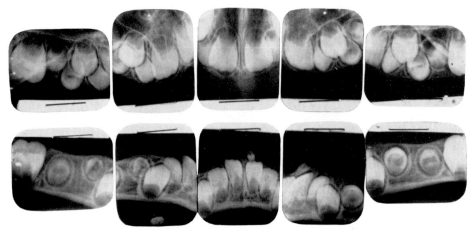

Fig. 81.—Boy, aged 4 years. Premature exfoliation of the deciduous dentition with root |a̱ retained. Well-marked calcification of the crowns of the unerupted second dentition.

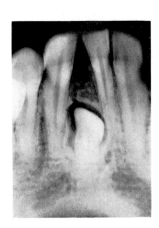

Fig. 82.—ɪ̱| unerupted. Not a common condition.

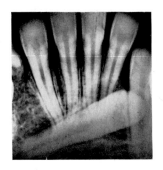

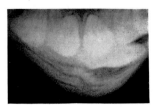

Fig. 83.—Boy, aged 13 years. 3̱| unerupted. The occlusal view shows the unerupted tooth lying buccally. Unilateral un- erupted canines are not as common as are the bilateral.

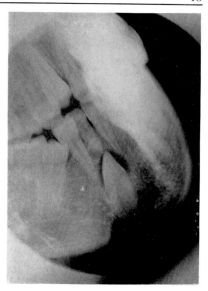

Fig. 84.—Girl, aged 13 years. 3| unerupted due to retained c̄| and a supernumerary tooth.

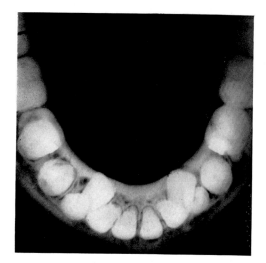

Fig. 85.—Boy, aged 15 years. 3̄|3̄ un-erupted, and both directed lingually. c̄|c̄ retained in situ.

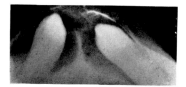

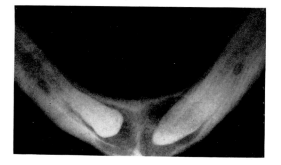

Fig. 86.—3̄|3̄ unerupted in edentulous patient. Impaction of the mandibular canine is a rare condition. The lower canines develop near the inferior border of the mandible and, when unerupted, are found deeply placed in the jaw.

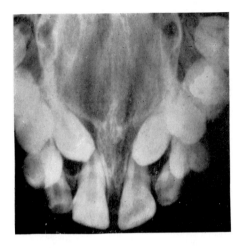

Fig. 87.—Girl, aged 10 years. 3|3 bilateral unerupted upper canine teeth. Lying at an angle to each other and directed mesially. Impaction may cause resorption of the roots and apices of the incisors.

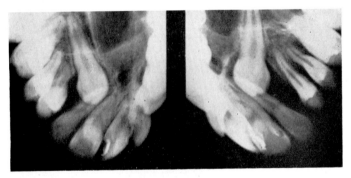

Fig. 88.—Topographical views of the unerupted 3|3 to show that they lie palatally. The upper canine teeth tend to erupt with some forward obliquity, more often with a palatal inclination than with a buccal slope.

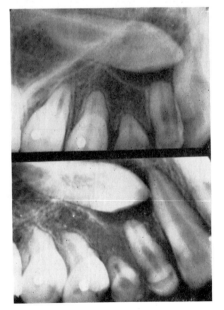

A

B

Fig. 89.—Parallax method to demonstrate the position of the unerupted canine 3|. A, the X-ray beam was directed at right angles to the canine region. B, as the X-ray tube moved to the left, the tip of the canine also moved in the same direction, and the tooth is therefore a greater distance from the tube, and lies on the palatal side.

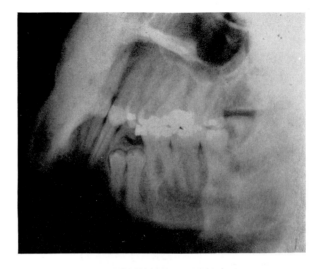

Fig. 90.—Man, aged 40 years. |45 unerupted. No apparent cause.

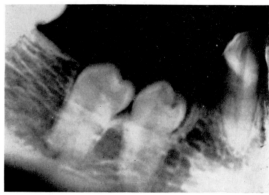

Fig. 91.—Man, aged 31 years. 54| unerupted. Have reached the alveolar margin, but appear to have been arrested.

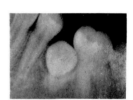

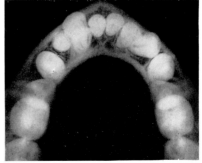

Fig. 92.—Girl, aged 12 years. 5|5 unerupted. The occlusal view shows that the unerupted teeth are directed lingually.

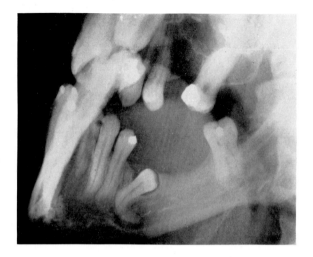

Fig. 93.—Man, aged 24 years. |5̄ unerupted and bent upon itself with the crown directed backwards.

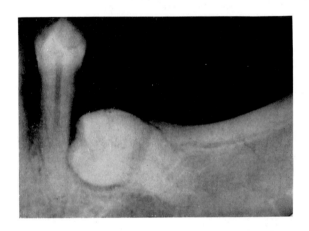

Fig. 94.—Female, aged 40 years. |5̄ unerupted and impacted against |4̄.

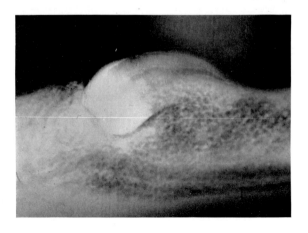

Fig. 95.—Woman, aged 46 years. |5̄ unerupted, lying at the alveolar margin with the root adopting an upward convex arch formation.

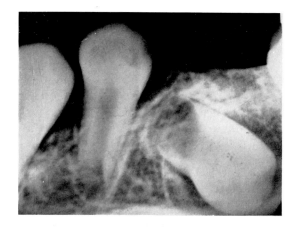

Fig. 96.—Boy, aged 10 years. $\overline{|5}$ unerupted and directed downwards and backwards.

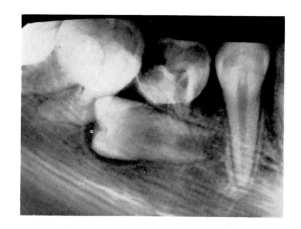

Fig. 97.—Girl, aged 13 years. $\overline{5|}$ unerupted with retained $\overline{e|}$.

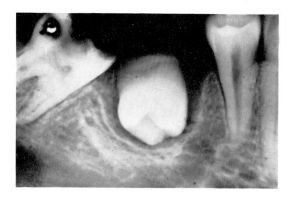

Fig. 98.—Boy, aged 16 years. Unerupted and completely inverted $\overline{5|}$. Inversion is an extremely rare condition.

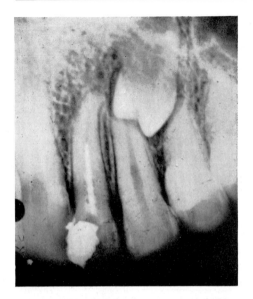

Fig. 99.—Girl, aged 19 years. |4 delayed eruption.

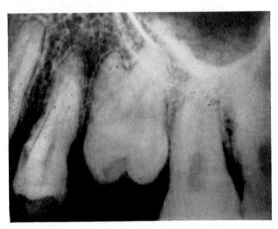

Fig. 100.—Man, aged 22 years. |5 delayed eruption.

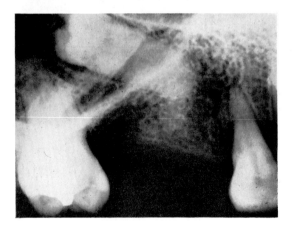

Fig. 101.—Woman, aged 43 years. 5| unerupted, lying beneath the floor of the right antrum, and directed upwards and backwards.

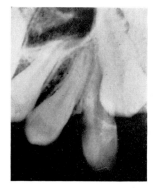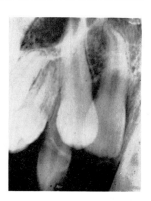

Fig. 102.—3| unerupted and transposed between unerupted 1| and fully erupted 2|.

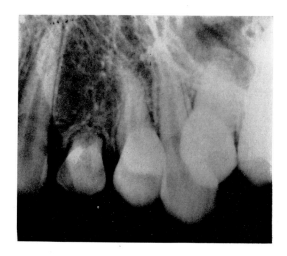

Fig. 103.—Transposed |3 between |4 and |5. |c retained.

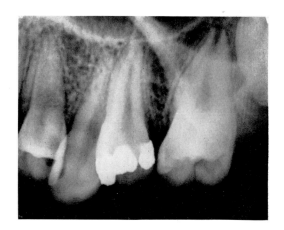

Fig. 104.—|3 transposed between |4 and |5.

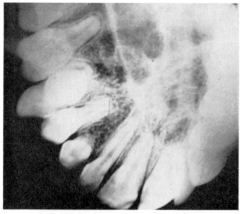

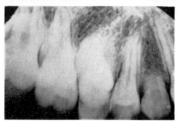

Fig. 105.—3| transposed labially between 4| and 5|. c| retained. 5| unerupted.

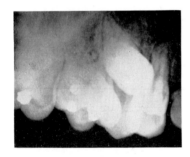

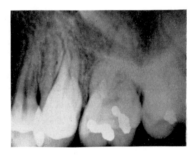

Fig. 106.—Girl, aged 13 years. Bilateral transposition 3|3 between 54|45.

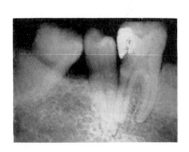

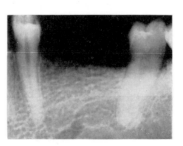

Fig. 107.—Woman, aged 30 years. 5| is transposed between 6| and 8|. On the left side there is a large gap between the premolars with |5 impacted against |8. This tooth also appears to be a transposed |5, and the intervening molar teeth have been lost.

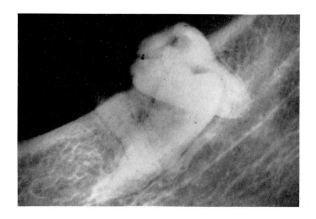

Fig. 108.—Woman, aged 34 years. $\overline{|5}$ unerupted has migrated backwards and become transposed between root $\overline{|7}$ and erupted $\overline{|8}$.

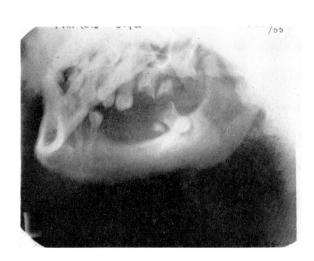

Fig. 109.—Woman, aged 25 years. $\overline{|5}$ unerupted has migrated backwards lying under retained root $\overline{|7}$ and impacted against root $\overline{|8}$.

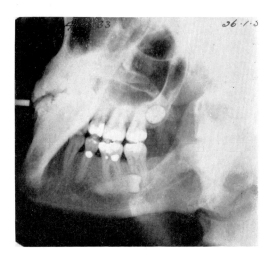

Fig. 110.—Woman, aged 33 years. Unerupted $\overline{|5}$ directed backwards and lying across roots $\overline{|6}$ and $\overline{|7}$.

SUBMERGED TEETH

The second deciduous molar tooth may be found below the plane of normal occlusion, especially in the lower jaw, and particularly when there is no successor.

It is still described as a submerged tooth, implying that it had erupted to its true position in the jaw, and that it had since become depressed or pushed below its original level. The modern accepted explanation is that during some stage in the growing period of the tooth and alveolus the periodontal membrane around the tooth is affected by infection or trauma. The injured membrane then undergoes a local necrosis or a fibroblastic degeneration, and is followed by subsequent new bone formation.

The osteoblastic reaction extends across from one or more points on the root to the bone of the socket wall and forms a bridge of bony union between them. In this way the tooth is tethered or anchored locally and is arrested in its centrifugal progress.

The partial ankylosis of the tooth to the bone causes retarded eruption, but the immediate and surrounding alveolar bone continues to grow in its vertical dimension, leaving the anchored tooth behind. The "submerged tooth" may be sited deep in the bone. The adjoining teeth continue in their elevation with the normal growth of the remaining part of the alveolus, and in the absence of a separating factor, tend to close over the low-lying anchored tooth.

The so-called "submergence" of the teeth is sometimes found in the second dentition, and here the teeth involved are generally the first permanent molars.

MALERUPTION AND IMPACTION

Maleruption and impaction of a tooth are attributed to various causes. In the former, the tooth assumes an abnormal position in the dental arch, whilst in the latter the tooth is in its true position, but is prevented from erupting by the presence of another tooth or tooth formation.

Trauma to the permanent tooth-germ is a common cause of maleruption. Equally as common is a delay or premature loss of a deciduous tooth. A retained root of the first dentition acts like a supernumerary, preventing the normal eruption of the under-lying tooth.

The third molar teeth are more frequently impacted than any other tooth and are classified according to the positions they adopt. Examples are shown in: (1) Vertical impaction. (2) Mesio-angular impaction. (3) Horizontal impaction. (4) Disto-angular impaction. (5) Transverse impaction.

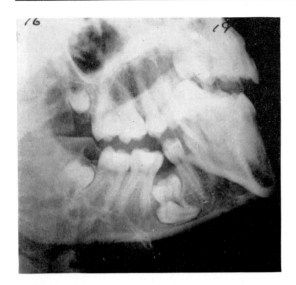

Fig. 111.—E⌋ submerged with un-erupted ⫠5⌋ lying horizontally and directed backwards.

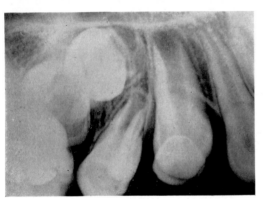

Fig. 112.—E⌋ submerged with unerupted 5⌋. 3⌋ unerupted.

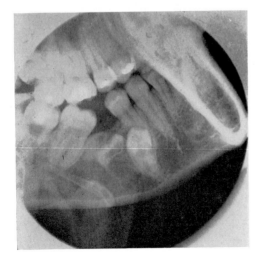

Fig. 113.—E⌋ submerged with ⫠5⌋ un-erupted and lying vertically.

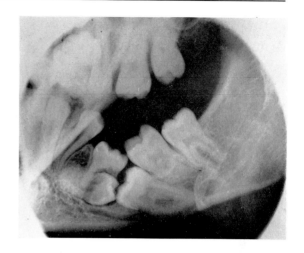

Fig. 114.—$\overline{6|}$ submerged. $\overline{|5}$ unerupted, directed backwards against the crown of the submerged $\overline{|6}$. $\overline{|E}$ retained and submerging.

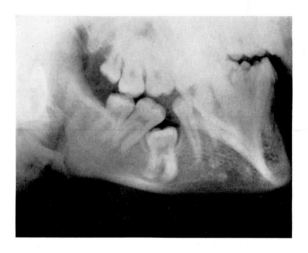

Fig. 115.—$\overline{6|}$ submerging as a result of pressure of inclining $\overline{7|}$.

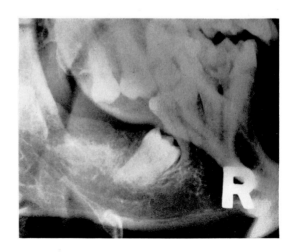

Fig. 116.—$\overline{6|}$ submerged after the extraction of $\overline{87|}$.

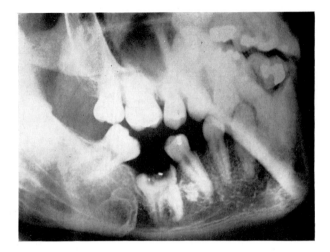

Fig. 117.—6̅| submerged. 7̅| extracted two years previously.

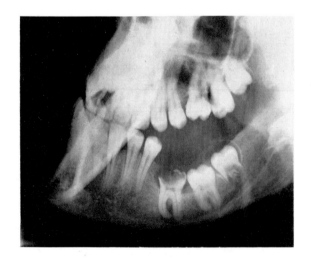

Fig. 118.—|6̅ submerged in an abscess area. |7̅8̅ unerupted.

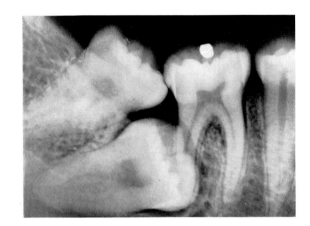

Fig. 119.—$\overline{7|}$ submerged by the tilting $\overline{8|}$ which is impacted against $\overline{6|}$.

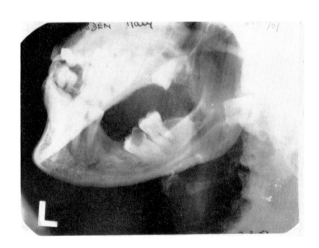

Fig. 120.—$\overline{|7}$ submerging from pressure of $\overline{|8}$. $\overline{|6}$ extracted a year previously.

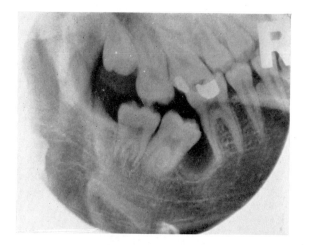

Fig. 121.—7| with follicular cyst being pushed downwards and mesially.

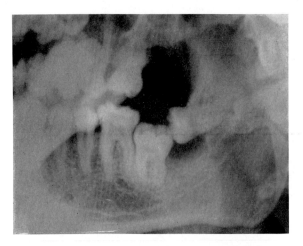

Fig. 122.—|7 submerging as a result of pressure from a horizontally impacted |8 and its large follicular cyst.

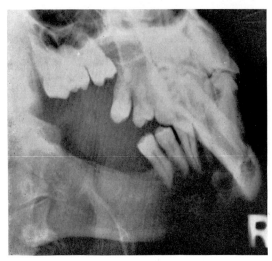

Fig. 123.—876| submerged.

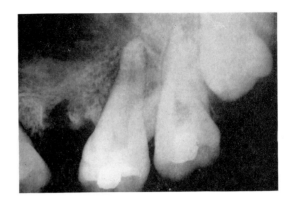

Fig. 124.—|8 vertical impaction. Tooth appears to be lying in a normal position, but is crowded against the roots of |7, and might eventually become impacted under the distal aspect of the crown of |7.

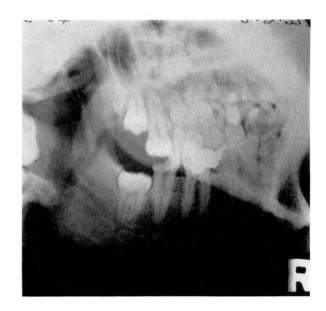

Fig. 125.— $\frac{8}{8}$| vertical impaction against the distal aspects of the $\frac{7}{7}$|. Distal part of the crown of $\overline{8|}$ is under the lower end of the anterior border of the ascending ramus.

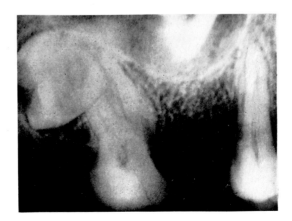

Fig. 126.—Disto-angular impaction. The upper third molar tooth is directed backwards and downwards.

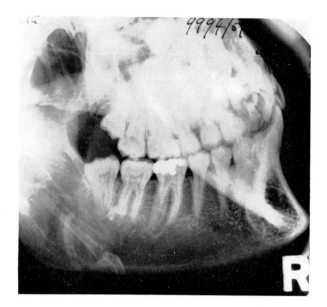

Fig. 127.—$\frac{8|}{8|}$ disto-angular impaction with crowns directed backwards.

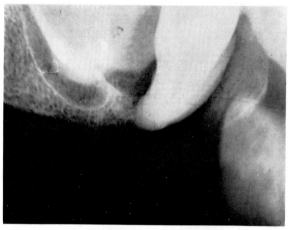

Fig. 128.—$|8$ disto-angular position with tooth inverted. The crown is directed upwards in the maxillary tuberosity, and the apices are at the alveolar border.

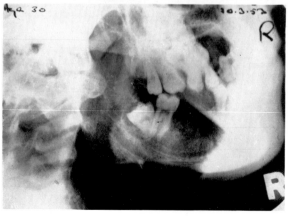

Fig. 129.—$\overline{8|}$ disto-angular impaction with the crown directed upwards and backwards and embedded in the lower part of the ascending ramus. The roots are pushed mesially against those of $\overline{7|}$.

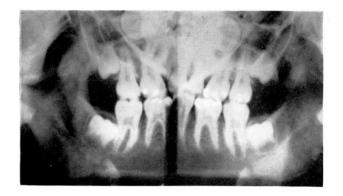

Fig. 130.—$\frac{8|8}{8|8}$ mesio-angular impaction. The impaction is against the middle third of the $\frac{7|7}{7|7}$.

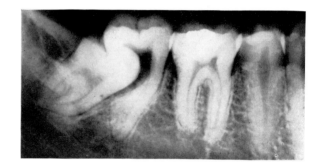

Fig. 131.—Mesio-angular impaction with erosion of distal part of $\overline{7|}$. Most frequent type of impaction.

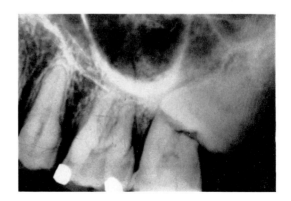

Fig. 132.—$|8$ mesio-angular impaction with resorption of the distal part of the roots of $|8$.

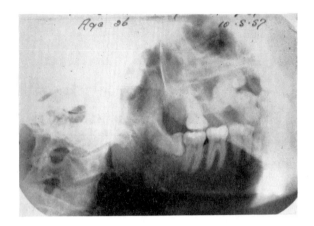

Fig. 133.—8̅| horizontal impaction against crown of 7̅|.

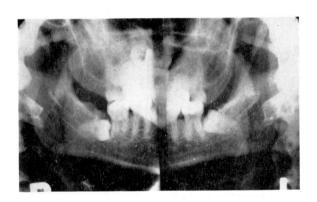

Fig. 134.—8̅|8̅ horizontal impaction against the terminal part of the roots of 7̅|7̅.

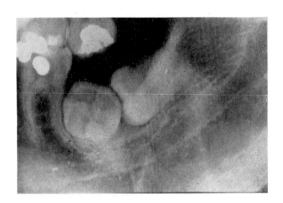

Fig. 135.—|8̅ horizontal impaction against unerupted |7̅. Horizontal impaction of the maxillary third molar teeth is rarely seen.

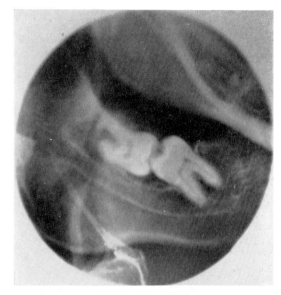

Fig. 136.—$\overline{8|}$ horizontal impaction (crown to crown) against unerupted $\overline{7|}$ which is directed backwards.

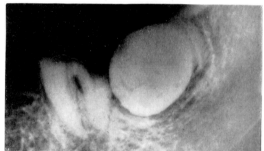

Fig. 137.—$\overline{|8}$ transverse impaction, probably a mesio-angular impaction deflected lingually and now lying transversely across the mandible.

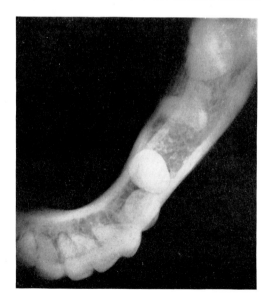

Fig. 138.—$\overline{|8}$ transverse impaction. Occlusal view of Fig. 137.

ANODONTIA

Complete anodontia in both dentitions is an extremely rare condition and is probably due to an endocrine imbalance. It is stated as being associated with deficiencies in the growth of the hair, nails, and sweat-glands.

In the absence of teeth, the alveolar bone shows poor and limited growth in height. Cases have been reported of the absence of all the permanent teeth following a full eruption of all the deciduous teeth. No other signs of ectodermal dysplasia are present in such circumstances, and the person is normal in all other respects.

Partial anodontia, particularly in the permanent dentition, is a comparatively common occurrence. The absence of one or more teeth is due to lack of development in the formative organs of that particular dentition. These deficiencies occur in any part of the dental arch, upper or lower, and may vary from the absence of a single tooth to a number of them, and are commonly symmetrical on both sides of the jaws.

Any of the teeth could be missing, but those rarely affected are the upper central incisors and the first two molars in the maxilla and mandible on either side. The absence of a permanent tooth is often associated with late retention of the deciduous tooth, which may itself become ankylosed.

5

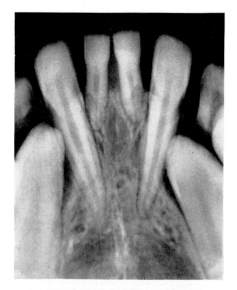

Fig. 139.—Child, aged 9 years. $\overline{1|1}$ absent.

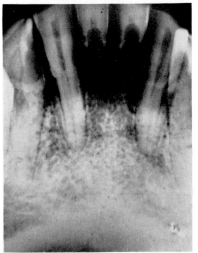

Fig. 140.—Child, aged 10 years. $\overline{1|1}$ absent.

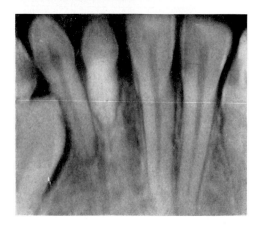

Fig. 141.—Child, aged 14 years. $\overline{21|}$ absent.

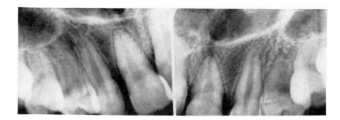

Fig. 142.—Child, aged 15 years. 2|2 absent.

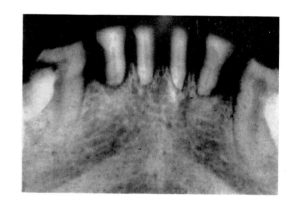

Fig. 143.—Child, aged 14 years. 21|12 absent.

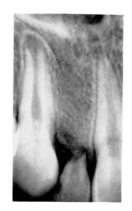
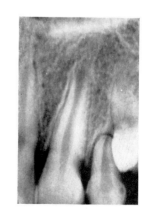

Fig. 144.—Child, aged 14 years. 2|2 absent.

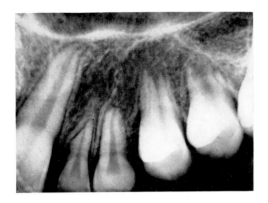

Fig. 145.—Child, aged 11 years. |3 absent.

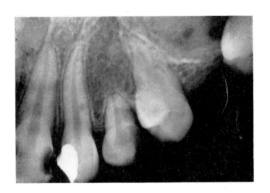

Fig. 146.—Girl, aged 13 years. |4 absent.

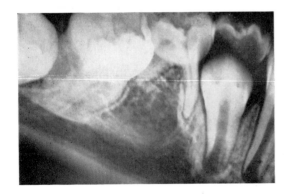

Fig. 147.—Girl, aged 9 years. 5| absent.

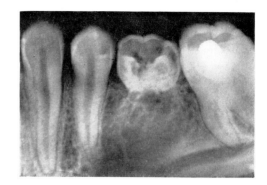

Fig. 148.—Girl, aged 13 years. $\overline{|5}$ absent.

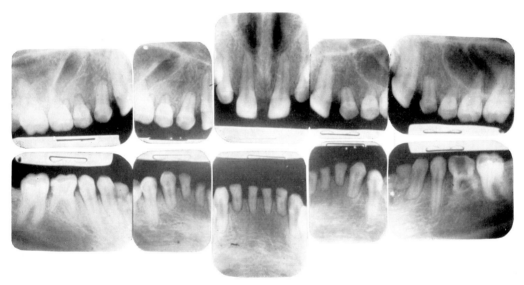

Fig. 149.—Boy, aged 10 years. $\dfrac{5432}{5\ 321}\Big|\dfrac{2345}{123\ 5}$ absent.

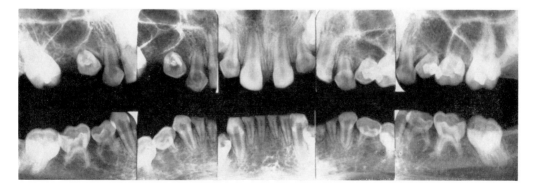

Fig. 150.—Girl, aged 10 years. $\dfrac{5432}{54321}\Big|\dfrac{2345}{12345}$ absent.

SUPERNUMERARY TEETH

Supernumerary teeth occur in both the deciduous and permanent dentitions in the upper and lower jaws. The only areas unaffected by additional teeth are the canine and the first and second molar regions.

The erupted supernumerary teeth are readily recognized on clinical examination. However, most of the unerupted supernumerary teeth are discovered during the course of routine X-ray examination. Their presence should be suspected if there is a gap or divergence between two permanent teeth, indicating delay in the eruption of the normal tooth by an obstructing supernumerary tooth.

An unerupted supernumerary tooth may cause rotation of immediate erupted teeth, tilting of these teeth, or their displacement in their arches. The majority of the supernumerary teeth are later in development and eruption than the permanent teeth.

Radiographically, the unerupted teeth may be identified as calcified crowns with undeveloped roots in dental crypts. Many appear with fully formed roots and emulate the teeth of the region in which they occur. Some are rudimentary in formation, but the majority, when erupted, adopt either a conical or tuberculated formation. The conical variety are the more common type, and the latter are rarely seen in the deciduous dentition. One often finds in the lateral incisor region in the upper jaw, supernumerary teeth fully erupted and identical in shape to the permanent teeth, which are known as supplemental teeth.

Supernumerary teeth may be multiple in the same patient, but if two or more are found in the same region they are not necessarily symmetrical in shape or direction. The position of supernumerary teeth varies considerably, not only as to their sites, but whether they lie palatally or buccally.

Occasionally, a follicular or dentigerous cyst is found in connexion with an unerupted supernumerary tooth. It is good practice to remove unerupted supernumerary teeth to overcome a delay in eruption of the normal tooth. In many instances, a retained supernumerary tooth may become impacted against a root of a permanent tooth and cause insidious resorption of that root.

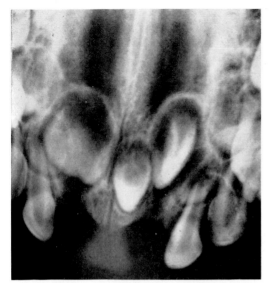

Fig. 151.—Boy, aged 18 months. 1|1 unerupted with an unerupted super-numerary tooth lying to the mesial side of |1. a|a were lost as a result of an accident.

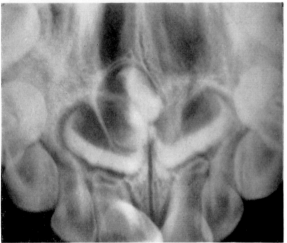

Fig. 152.—Infant, aged 1 year 7 months. 21|12 unerupted with unerupted supernumerary lying mesial to 1|.

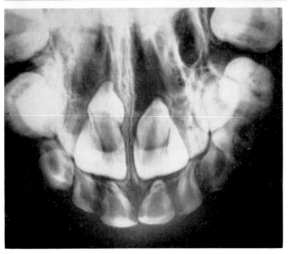

Fig. 153.—Boy, aged 4 years. 321|123 unerupted, with unerupted supernumeraries lying on either side of the middle line on the palatal side of 1|1.

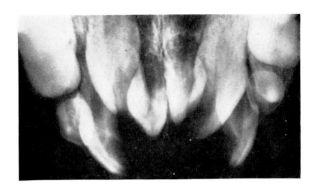

Fig. 154.—Patient, aged 5½ years. 1|1 unerupted, with an unerupted supernumerary lying on either side of the middle line, and obstructing the eruption of the upper central incisors.

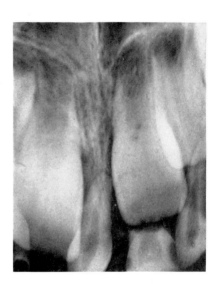

Fig. 155.—Patient, aged 5 years. 1|1 unerupted, with an erupted supernumerary in the midline. a| exfoliated a year previously.

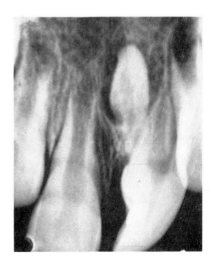

Fig. 156.—Boy, aged 7 years. 1|1 fully erupted with inverted supernumerary in |1 region. |1 rotated. Probably due to the presence of unerupted supernumerary.

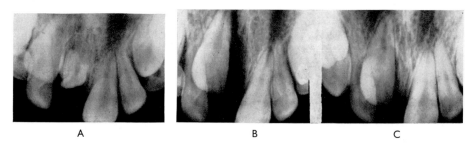

A   B   C

Fig. 157.—Patient, aged 9 years. **A**, unerupted supernumerary in the right upper central incisor region, obstructing the eruption of 1|. **B, C**, show progress of eruption of 1| after the extraction of the unerupted supernumerary.

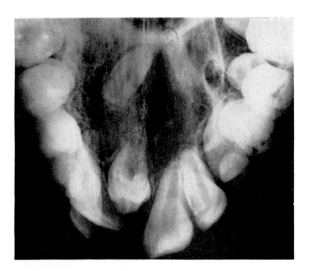

Fig. 158.—Patient, aged 9 years. Two unerupted supernumerary teeth lying in the midline of the palate, one in the upper incisor region, and the other in the transverse premolar line.

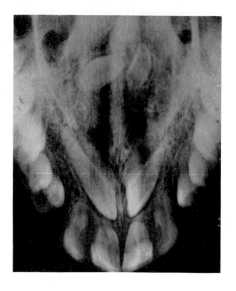

Fig. 159.—Patient, aged 21 years. Two unerupted supernumeraries lying on either side of the midline in the transverse molar plane. 3|3 unerupted and directed mesially to each other.

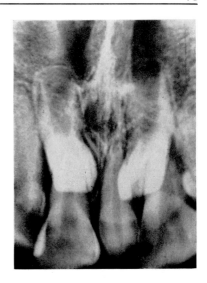

Fig. 160.—Patient, aged 11 years. Three supernumeraries in the upper incisor region, one erupted in the middle line, and two unerupted and lying palatally to the 1|1.

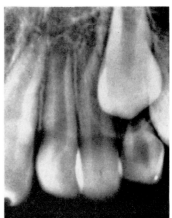

Fig. 161.—Patient, aged 9 years. Supplemental erupted tooth in |2 region. |3 unerupted.

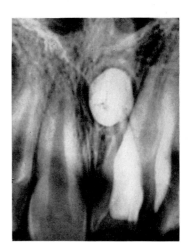

Fig. 162.—Patient, aged 11 years. Unerupted supernumerary in |1 region. Unerupted supplemental tooth in |2 region.

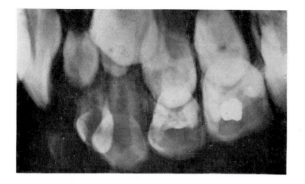

Fig. 163.—Patient, aged 8 years. Unerupted supplemental tooth in the |2 region. |12345 unerupted.

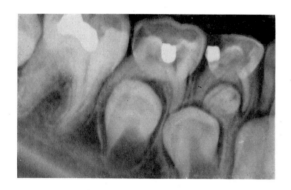

Fig. 164.—Patient, aged 9 years. Unerupted supernumerary in 4| region. 543| unerupted.

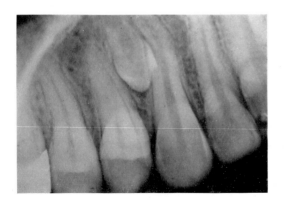

Fig. 165.—Patient, aged 17 years. Unerupted supernumerary between 3| and 4|.

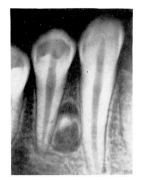
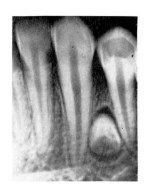

Fig. 166.—Patient, aged 18 years. Unerupted supernumeraries in $\overline{4|4}$ region.

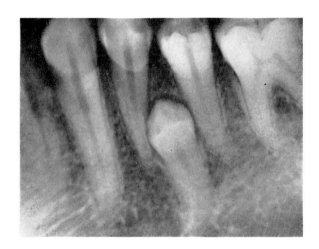

Fig. 167.—Unerupted supernumerary between $\overline{|4}$ and $\overline{|5}$.

Fig. 168.—Patient, aged 21 years. Unerupted supernumerary in $\overline{4|}$ region and an unerupted supernumerary between $\overline{|5}$ and $\overline{|6}$.

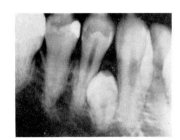
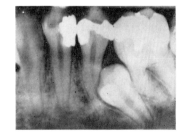

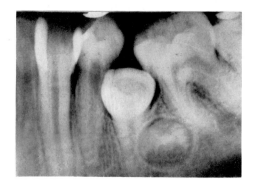

Fig. 169.—Unerupted supernumerary tooth in $\overline{5}$ region. $\overline{5}$ unerupted.

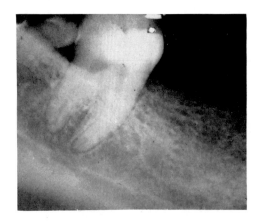

Fig. 170.—Unerupted rudimentary supernumerary tooth in $\overline{8|}$ region.

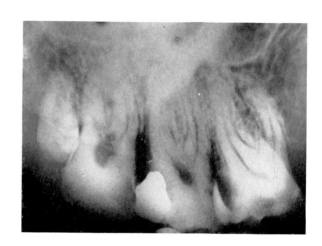

Fig. 171.—Unerupted rudimentary supernumerary tooth in 8| region.

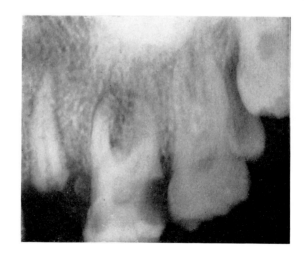

Fig. 172.—Unerupted rudimentary supernumerary tooth between |7 and unerupted |8.

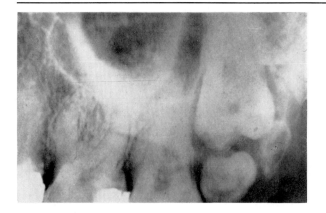

Fig. 173.—Unerupted rudimentary supernumerary tooth lying below unerupted |8.

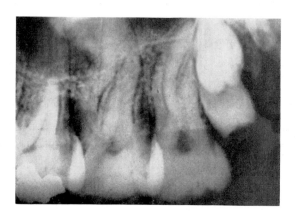

Fig. 174.—Two unerupted rudimentary supernumerary teeth lying behind the |8.

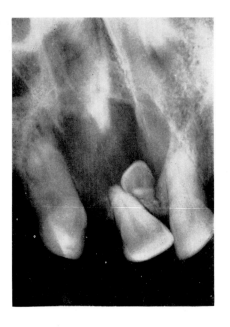

Fig. 175.—Unerupted supernumerary tooth in the 1| region, associated with a large dentigerous cyst.

IV.—Anomalies in Tooth Formation

  1. Roots.
  2. Crowns.
      a. Malformation.
      b. Hypoplasia.
      c. Amelogenesis imperfecta.
      d. Dentinogenesis imperfecta.
  3. Pulp.
      a. Pulp stones.
      b. Obliteration of the canal.

Anomalies in Tooth Formation

DEFECTS in the development and growth of the teeth may affect the roots, the crowns, or the pulp.

1. Roots.—The roots may be stunted or elongated with no apparent underlying cause. Single-rooted teeth may be bifurcated or angulated, multi-rooted teeth fused (commonly in two rooted molars), whilst extra roots may be found in all teeth of the permanent dentition except the upper and lower incisors.

2. Crowns.—

a. Malformed Crowns may be abnormally wide or unusually narrow, and occasionally the canines may be bifid. The molar teeth may show variations in their cusp formation. Cases have been reported of grotesque malformations of the crown with correspondingly peculiar root formations, but the most common departures are conical or peg-top shaped crowns. Some of the teeth show peculiar erosion of the crown and many adopt club or mushroom-like formations.

b. Hypoplasia of the Enamel is rarely seen in the first dentition. It is frequently met with in the permanent teeth.

Postnatal hypoplasia is said to be due to infection or lack of certain vitamins. Both produce a retardation of calcification of the teeth.

When a single tooth is affected it usually follows upon trauma or infection. The involvement of a number of teeth is associated with an hereditary factor and grouped under the classification of (*c*) *amelogenesis imperfecta*, or (*d*) *dentinogenesis imperfecta*.

In the former the dentine shows marked disturbances of formation, but the enamel is normal. The roots of the teeth are shortened and the root canals obliterated. In the latter, much of the enamel of the crown is missing, but the dentine formation is unaltered.

3. Pulp.—Deposition of calcium in the pulp may be seen as (*a*) pulp stones, or (*b*) diffuse calcification in the canals. Pulp stones are usually found in the coronal part of the pulp chamber and do not obliterate the canal.

The stones are found in both dentitions and there is much literature covering their aetiology, with a division of opinion as to the traumatic and physiological relationships. Only 15 per cent of pulp stones are sufficiently large to be visible radiographically, and they are found more frequently with increasing age. Occasionally one finds pulp stones occurring in both dentitions concurrently, with the condition observed in unerupted teeth.

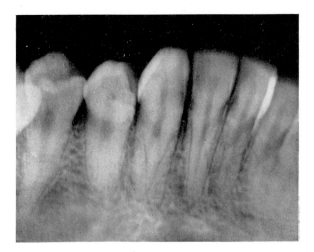

Fig. 176.—$\overline{3}|$ two-rooted. The canine is not as frequently affected as the premolars or the bicuspids.

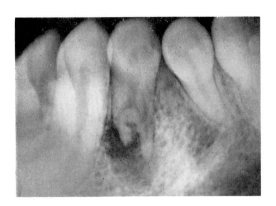

Fig. 177.—$\overline{|4}$ two-rooted with a superimposed peri-apical abscess.

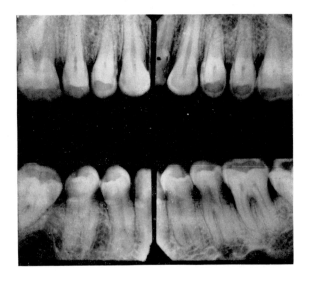

Fig. 178.—All the premolars in both jaws have two roots. This is not a rare occurrence.

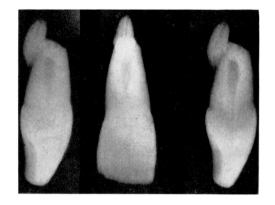

Fig. 179.—|3 dilacerated. This type of deformity is often associated with a traumatic history in the early stages of tooth development.

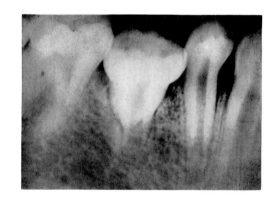

Fig. 180.—5| mushroom formation of the crown often described as a "club foot" shape. This is subject to impaction.

Fig. 181.—2| serrated incisive edge.

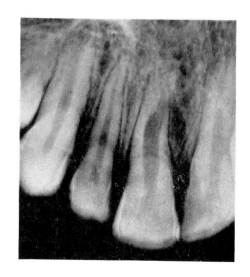

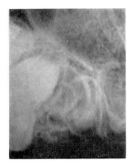
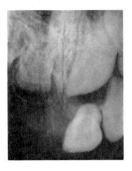

Fig. 182.—Boy, aged 5 years, with history of trauma. 3̲2̲1̲| unerupted. Hypoplasia, arrested development of crown and root. c̲b̲a̲| early loss. |1 appears normal.

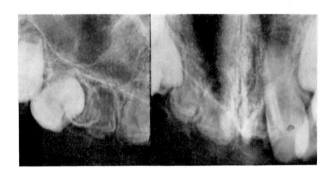

Fig. 183.—Boy, aged 9 years. Arrested development and hypocalcification of 3̲2̲1̲|1̲ .

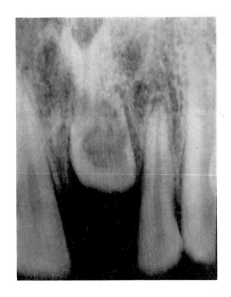

Fig. 184.—Male, aged 23 years. |1 unerupted. Hypoplasia and non-formation of root.

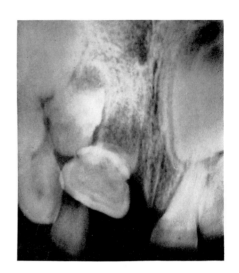

Fig. 185.—Boy, aged 5 years. 1| partially erupted with hypoplastic crown. 2| unerupted. Deformed hypoplastic crown.

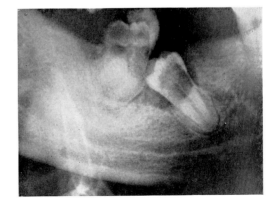

Fig. 186.—Patient, aged 42 years. 6| fully erupted. Hypoplasia of the crown. 5| unerupted and impacted against 6| with hypoplasia.

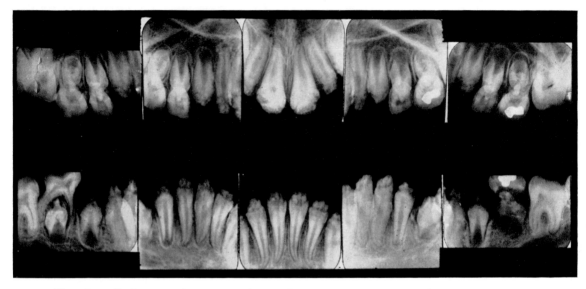

Fig. 187.—Patient, aged 9 years. Generalized amelogenesis imperfecta. Both dentitions are affected. The unerupted canines and premolars show marked hypoplasia, but the roots and pulp canals are normal.

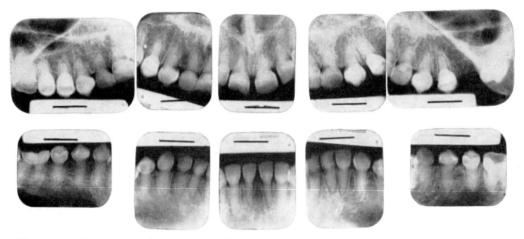

Fig. 188.—Patient, aged 18 years. Dentinogenesis imperfecta with opalescent dentine. This condition is usually hereditary. *Crowns*, Enamel of poor quality. *Roots*, Deficient root development. *Pulp chamber and canals*, Small and almost entirely obliterated, due to calcification of the pulp. Marked radiolucency around the root apices.

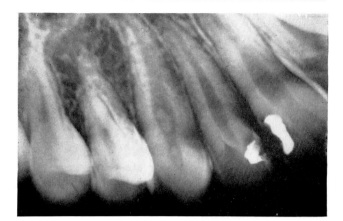

Fig. 189.—3| pulp stones in dilated pulp canal.

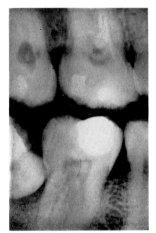

Fig. 190.—Pulp stones in the pulp chamber of the upper and lower molar teeth.

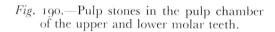

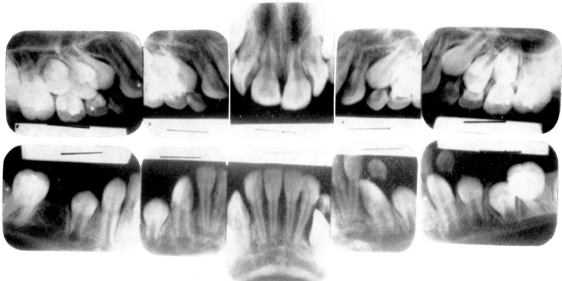

Fig. 191.—Pulp stones in the teeth of both dentitions. Pulp stones are seen in the canals of the partially erupted and unerupted teeth.

V.—Calcified Odontomes

1. Geminated.
2. Compound composite.
3. Compound complex.
4. Dilated.
5. Cystic.
6. Enamel pearls.
7. Dens in dente.
8. Cementoma.

Calcified Odontomes

Odontogenic Tumours

A CALCIFIED odontome results from an aberration of the whole tooth-germ and may contain varying combinations of enamel, dentine, cementum, pulp, and fibrous tissue. Each conglomeration is surrounded by a periodontal structure and an outer containing wall equivalent to the lamina dura. It may develop into a cystic condition. Odontomes may occur in any part of the maxilla or mandible.

The following types are differentiated:—

1. Geminated Odontome.—This is a fairly frequent occurrence and is a fusion of two or several, more or less well-formed teeth along any part of their formation.

All degrees of union may be identified, some with a common pulp chamber and separate roots, or vice versa.

These odontomes are more common in the deciduous dentition when the central and lateral incisors are involved. The third molar is the tooth usually affected in the permanent dentition.

2. Compound Composite Odontome.—This takes the form of a cluster of several denticles, rudimentary teeth, or discrete masses of dental tissue. They are seen at all ages. In early life they may prevent or impede normal eruption of teeth of the second dentition, and interfere with the alinement of neighbouring teeth, causing displacement and promoting migration of the unerupted tooth from its true position.

3. Compound Complex Odontome.—This entity consists of an irregular, un-organized, amorphous mass of the enamel, dentine, and cementum with a considerable proportion of bone. It bears little or no resemblance to the shape of the tooth. Radiographically, it simulates an area of sclerosis or even an osteoma, and may appear in edentulous regions in the premolar or molar mandibular sites. There is no sharply demarcated edge or any signs of a fibrous capsule. Some of them are found to be composed almost entirely of dentine and are then referred to as dentinomas.

4. Dilated Odontome.—These are rare conditions. The crown and root of an affected tooth show a marked internal enlargement and outer expansion.

5. Cystic Odontome.—The fibrous encapsulated compound or composite odontomes may be contained within a cystic wall with fluid. Similarly to ordinary cysts they enlarge slowly, and eventually produce expansion of the bone with asymmetry of the face.

6. Enamel Pearls, Enamel Drops, Enameloma.—This is a simple form of an odontome. It is a dense, superposed enamel bud external to the tooth surface, generally seen in multi-rooted teeth at their site of bifurcation. Some of these have been described as containing a core of pulp tissue formation extending from a main root of the parent tooth. These should be regarded as supernumerary odontomes.

7. Dens in Dente.—This formation results from an invagination during the development stage of the tooth. Ordinarily, they are found in the pulp canal. The coronal type are common in the upper permanent lateral incisor teeth and the radicular variety are more often seen in the molar teeth.

8. Cementoma.—This is an odontome of cementum and occurs as a rounded mass at the apex of a vital tooth. It is not produced by abnormal development of a tooth-germ, but forms after the root itself has been formed, and arises from the apical part of the dental follicle or from the mature periodontal membrane.

It should not be confused with hypercementosis, which is bulbous or fusiform in shape, and conforms to the general outline of the root. It has also been described as a form of peri-apical osteofibrosis and attributed to traumatic occlusion or other types of trauma. It may arise through calcification in a fibrous odontome.

In its initial stage of soft tissue formation it cannot cast a shadow on an X-ray film. When the growth is complete, the cementum presents a homogeneous, spherical, opaque mass attached to the apex of the tooth.

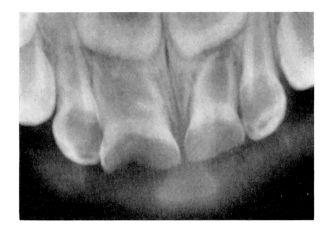

Fig. 192.—Patient, aged 22 months. a|a. Both the upper temporary central incisors are geminated.

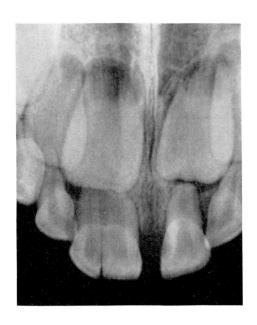

Fig. 193.—Patient, aged 5 years. a|. This shows fusion with a supernumerary.

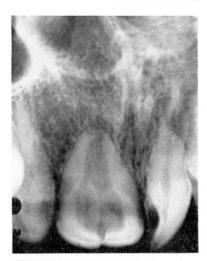

Fig. 194.—Patient, aged 7 years. Geminated 1| with a double pulp chamber, but single root canal.

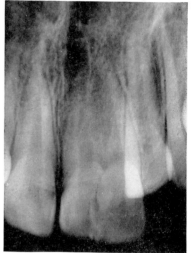

Fig. 195.—Patient, aged 9 years. |1. The gemination is of the fused type, probably to a supernumerary, each with its own pulp canal and chamber.

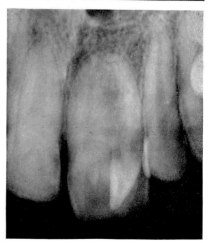

Fig. 196.—Patient, aged 12 years. |1. Geminated tooth with a dens in dente.

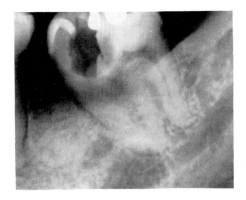

Fig. 197.—Patient, aged 40 years. |8.
Geminated.

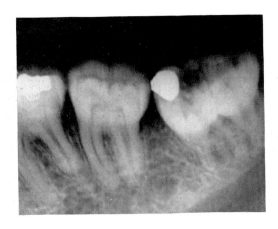

Fig. 198.—Patient, aged 21 years. |8.
Geminated, with supplemental molar.

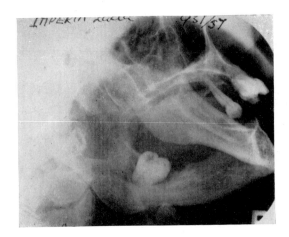

Fig. 199.—Patient, aged 48 years.
8|. Geminated 8| in edentulous lower
jaw.

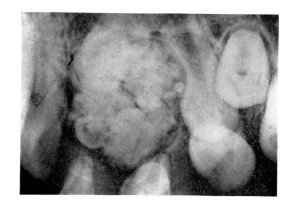

Fig. 200.—Patient, aged 9 years. |2. Compound composite odontome. At operation was found to be encapsulated, and contained a fully formed lateral tooth, and innumerable small denticles.

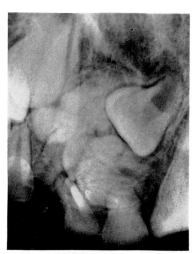

Fig. 201.—Patient, aged 9 years. 21|. The central and lateral incisors are prevented from erupting by this odontome.

Fig. 202.—Patient, aged 16 years. 54|. Composite odontome in the 54| region.

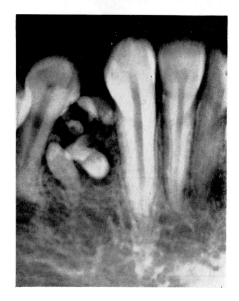

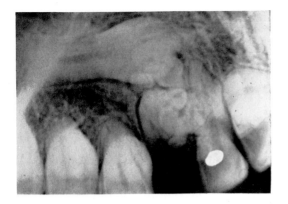

Fig. 203.—Patient, aged 20 years. Composite odontome impeding the eruption of 3|, which is lying horizontally high in the alveolar process of the maxilla.

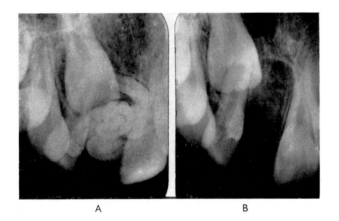

A   B

Fig. 204.—Patient, aged 10 years. A, Obstructed eruption of 1| by the compound composite odontome in this region. B, Advancing eruption of 1| after the removal of the odontome.

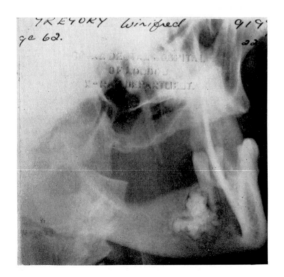

Fig. 205.—Patient, aged 62 years. Compound composite odontome in $\overline{54|}$ region, discovered during routine examination.

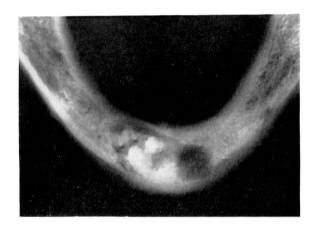

Fig. 206.—Patient, aged 53 years. Occlusal view showing compound composite odontome in an edentulous patient who complained of an ill-fitting denture.

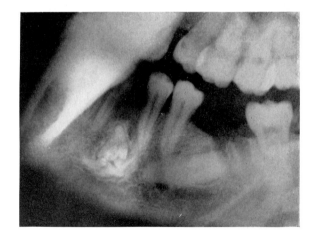

Fig. 207.—Patient, aged 30 years. Composite odontome in $\overline{|3}$ region causing migration of the $\overline{|3}$ backwards. It became impacted against $\overline{|6}$, which was eroded and had to be extracted.

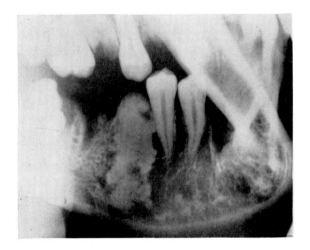

Fig. 208.—Compound complex odontome lying vertically in $\overline{6|}$ region and extending above the alveolar margin.

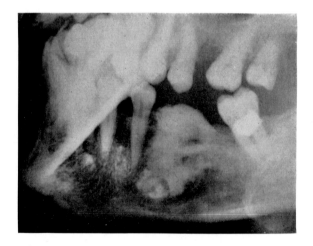

Fig. 209.—Another example of a compound complex odontome also vertical in position. No radiographic signs of encapsulation.

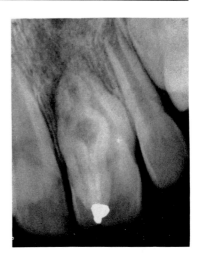

Fig. 210.—Dilated odontome. Patient, aged 9 years. |1. The whole of the tooth shows a marked enlargement or expansion.

Fig. 211.—Cystic odontome. Patient, aged 56 years. Cystic complex odontome in 8| region.

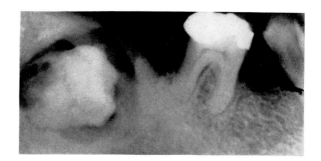

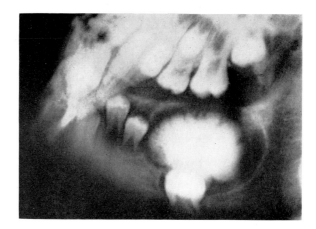

Fig. 212.—Patient, aged 10 years. Large cystic complex odontome in the left mandibular region obstructing the eruption of |6, which is completely submerged and penetrating the lower border of the mandible.

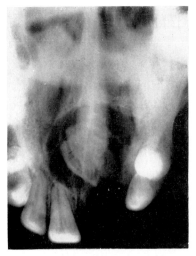

Fig. 213.—Occlusal view of large cystic compound odontome in the |12 region, and extending across the midline suture.

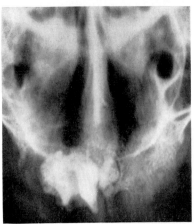

Fig. 214.—Occlusal view of a cystic composite odontome in 321| region which was thought to be a retained root.

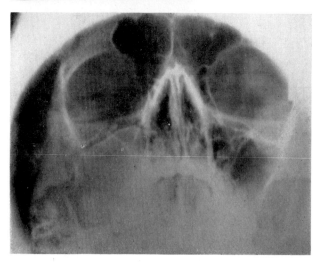

Fig. 215.—Patient, aged 16 years. A cystic odontome on the right side invaginating and occupying the whole of the right antrum. The denticles are seen on the outer wall of the antrum in its lower posterior half, which is eroded.

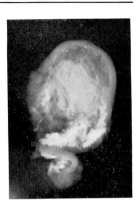

Fig. 216.—A radiograph of the enucleated cystic odontome in *Fig.* 215 after removal.

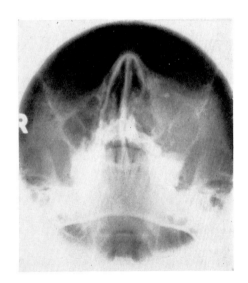

Fig. 217.—Patient, aged 14 years. Cystic odontome occupying the whole of the left antrum. The outer wall is expanded and bulging outwards, and there are two rudimentary teeth in the region of the floor of the right orbit, which is being pushed upwards and inwards.

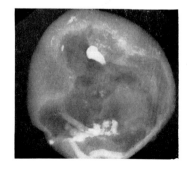

Fig. 218.—Patient, aged 14 years. Radiograph of the enucleated cystic odontome in *Fig.* 217.

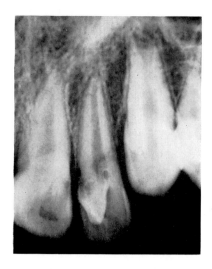

Fig. 219.—Patient, aged 11 years. |2. Dens in dente with apex closed.

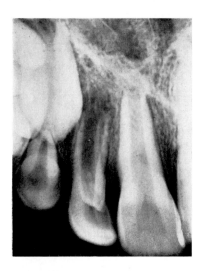

Fig. 220.—Patient, aged 8 years. 2|. Dens in dente with apex open.

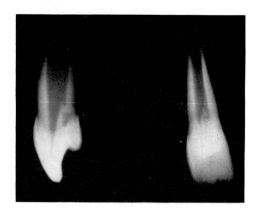

Fig. 221.—Patient, aged 8 years. Lateral and labial radiographs of dens in dente. 2|.

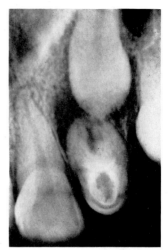

Fig. 222.—Patient, aged 13 years. Dens in dente replacing the normal |2 with |3 unerupted.

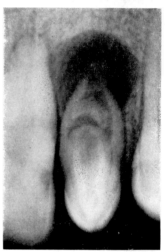

Fig. 223.—Dens in dente replacing |2 with apical abscess.

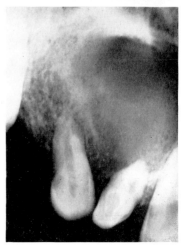

Fig. 224.—Patient, aged 22 years. 2|. Dens in dente 2| with large odontogenic cyst.

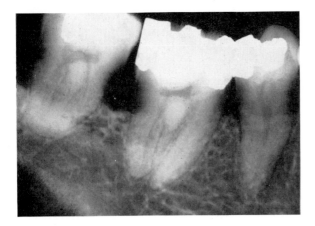

Fig. 225.—Enameloma. Structureless radio-opaque shadow situated at the bifurcation of the roots of 6̄|.

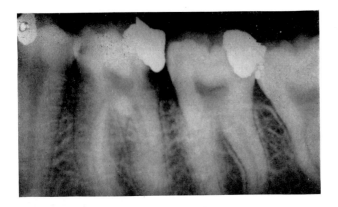

Fig. 226.—Enameloma at the bifurcation of the roots of |6̄. Complete absence of a pulp chamber.

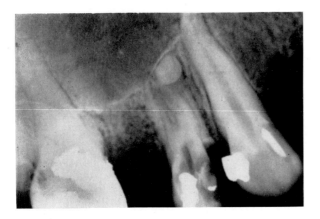

Fig. 227.—Cementoma. Rounded radio-opaque structure attached to the apex of the tooth, showing that the mass is within the tip of the socket.

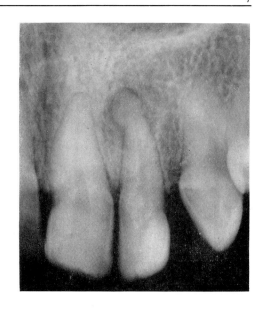

Fig. 228.—Cementoma. Another example of a rounded radio-opaque structure attached to the apex of the tooth.

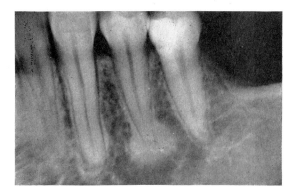

Figs. 229, 230.—Cementoma. The deposit of cementum has formed outside the socket. This appearance is sometimes described as peri-apical osteofibrosis where bone destruction has been replaced by fibrous tissue and cementum formation.

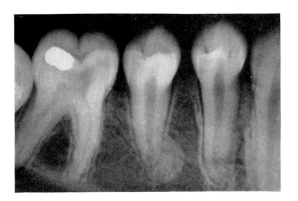

VI.—SALIVARY CALCULI

Salivary Calculi

CALCAREOUS deposits are found in the mouth either in association with the teeth or the salivary glands.

1. Dental Calculi.—

a. Tartar. Supragingival Calculus.—Deposition of calcium salts on the crowns of the teeth from the cervix to the cutting edge is common. There may be some connexion with secretion from the salivary glands. In the upper jaw the molar teeth, on their buccal surface near the orifice of Stensen's duct, are frequently affected. The lower incisor teeth on their lingual surface are in close approximation to the orifices of the submaxillary and sublingual glands.

Tartar deposits, although a frequent cause of gingival inflammation, are not necessarily associated with parodontal disease, alveolar recession, and 'pocketing'.

b. Seruminal Calculus. Subgingival Calculus.—This form of deposit is always associated with marginal gingivitis and forms in the pockets of parodontal disease.

2. Salivary Stones. (Sialolithiasis.)—The formation of calculi can take place either in the gland itself or in its duct. Stones may pass forward from the gland and remain stationary in the duct.

Salivary calculi in the parotid and sublingual glands are relatively rare, but are commonly found in the submaxillary gland and duct.

The stones vary considerably in size, shape, and number. Those located in the gland are usually large, rounded, or nodular, and homogeneous in density, while those found in the salivary duct are elongated or fusiform in the lumen of the duct. In many cases the concretions within the submaxillary duct tend to disintegrate or fracture and the X-ray picture shows a number of opacities in line in the path of the duct.

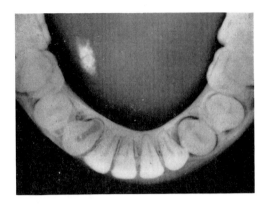

Fig. 231.—Calculus in right sub-maxillary duct on the lingual aspect of 5̄|.

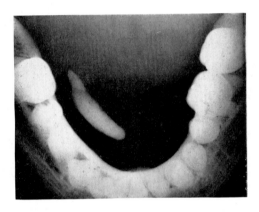

Fig. 232.—Elongated fusiform calculus situated in the anterior half of the left sub-maxillary duct. The concretion has adapted its conformation to the lumen of the duct.

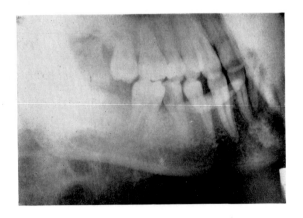

Fig. 233.—External oblique view of *Fig.* 232. The shadow of the salivary calculus has been projected upwards by the increased angulation of the X-ray beam.

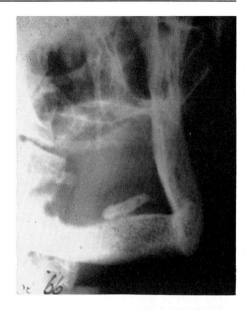

Fig. 234.—Extra-oral oblique lateral view showing the upward projection of the salivary calculus in an edentulous patient.

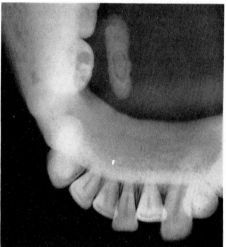

Fig. 235.—The elongated shadow of the calculus in the anterior part of the submaxillary gland shows an internal nucleus, around which the calcium deposit has formed.

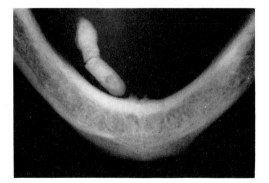

Fig. 236.—Occlusal view of Fig. 234 demonstrating a fracture across the middle of the calculus.

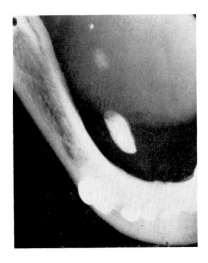

Fig. 237.—Fracture of the calculus in the right submaxillary duct with wide separation of the distal fragment from the main forward mass.

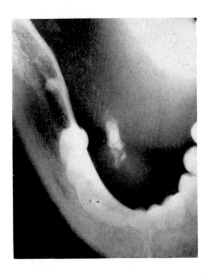

Fig. 238.—Fracture and fragmentation of the right salivary calculus with "kite-tail" disposition of the fragments in the duct.

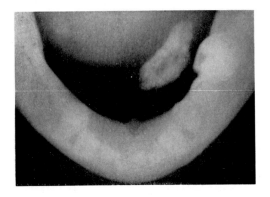

Fig. 239.—Irregular large calcareous mass-formation of a salivary calculus in the anterior part of the left submaxillary duct.

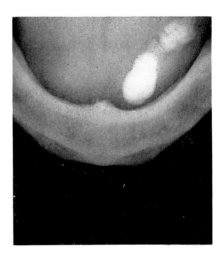

Fig. 240.—Bulbous salivary calculus at the proximal end of the left submaxillary duct obstructing the flow of the salivary secretion with progressive additional deposition behind it.

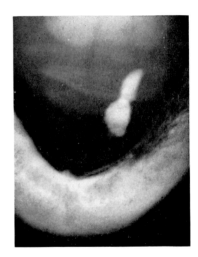

Fig. 241.—Salivary calculus in the proximal part of the left submaxillary duct with secondary inflammatory rarefaction of the lingual aspect of the left mandible.

Fig. 242.—Left sublingual calculus.

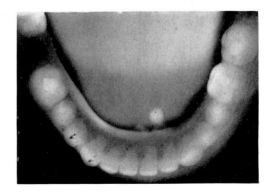

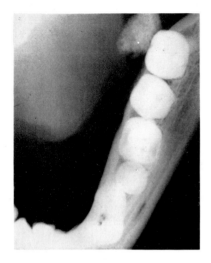

Fig. 243.—Occlusal view, demonstrating a calcareous deposit in the left submaxillary gland. The shadow is seen lying in the floor of the mouth on the lingual aspect of $\overline{|8}$.

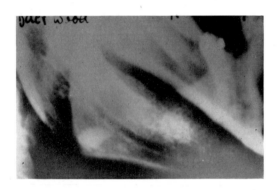

Fig. 244.—External oblique view, showing the shadow of a salivary calculus in the submaxillary gland superimposed upon the angle of the jaw.

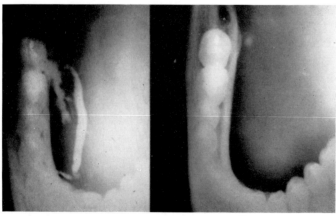

A   B

Fig. 245.—A, Occlusal view, showing a small calculus in the floor of the mouth lying on the lingual aspect of the last left lower molar tooth. B, Sialogram showing the opaque fluid in the left submaxillary duct. The duct is dilated due to the partial obstruction of the calculus. Some of the opaque medium has managed to trickle into the gland.

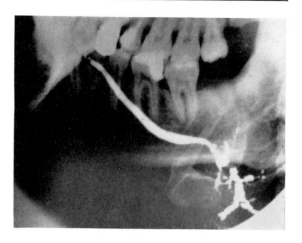

Fig. 246.—External oblique view of Fig. 245 showing the dilated left submaxillary duct.

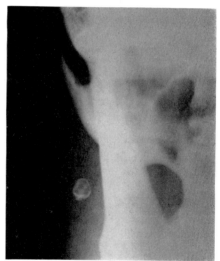

Fig. 247.—Large calculus in the right parotid gland.

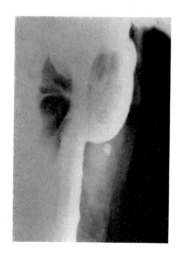

Fig. 248.—Calculus in the left parotid gland.

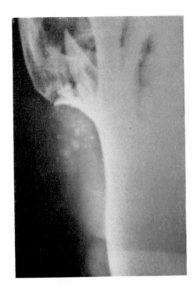

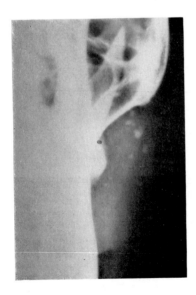

Figs. 249, 250.—Multiple small calculi in both
    parotid glands of the same patient.

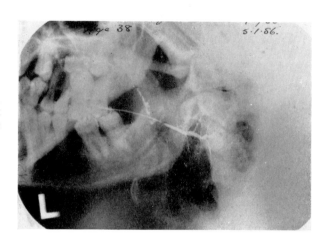

Fig. 251.—Sialogram of Fig. 250. Note dilatation of Stensen's duct in an attempt to overcome the obstruction of the calculi.

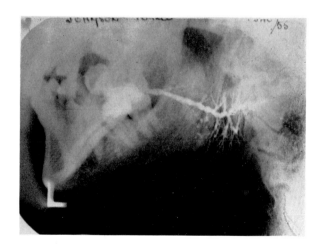

Fig. 252.—Sialogram of the left parotid duct with dilatation and segmentation.

PART II

INFLAMMATORY AND TRAUMATIC LESIONS
OF TEETH AND JAWS

Tooth Concussion

DIRECT violence to a tooth causes a jarring or impaction of the tooth against the socket wall. The intervening periodontal membrane at the very apex may be bruised. The resultant injury depends upon the severity of the concussion, and varies from the rupture of a few small capillaries to extravasation of blood and the formation of small hæmatomata in and around the apex of the tooth.

The following radiographic changes have been observed after concussion of a tooth:—

1. Changes in the periodontal membrane.
2. Hæmorrhagic complications.
3. Pulp reaction.
4. Developmental interference.
5. Resorption of the apex of the tooth.
6. Hypercementosis.
7. Bone reaction.
8. Ankylosis at the apex.
9. Superimposed infection.

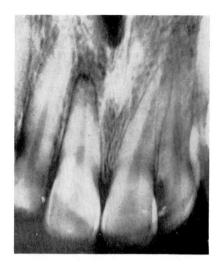

Fig. 253.—Patient, aged 19 years. Traumatic apical periodontitis. Received an accidental blow six days previously. Crown of 1| shows no evidence of caries or fracture. Slight thickening and irregularity of the apical periodontal membrane shadow. No signs of erosion or break in the continuity of the lamina dura.

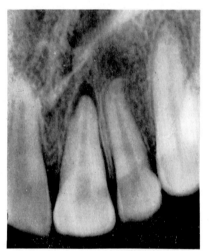

Fig. 254.—Patient, aged 15 years. Apical hæmatoma. Received a closed-fisted punch on mouth about four weeks previously. Relatively large black area at apex of |1. The injured tooth will probably lose its vitality and become prey to an added infection.

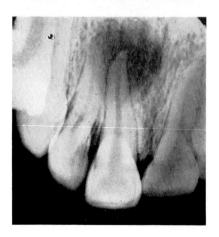

Fig. 255.—Patient, aged 24 years. Encapsulated hæmatoma. Ran into a lamp-post about three months previously. Large circular black area, radiating from the apex of 1| and overlying the apical half of the root and the bone beyond, with an equal radius. Tooth vital. The apical periodontal membrane and lamina dura show no abnormality. No bony porosis outside the socket.

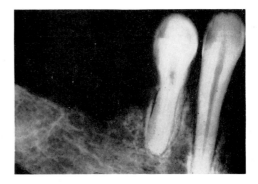

Fig. 256.—Patient, aged 43 years. Calcification of the pulp. Fall on the right jaw over three years previously. Obliteration of the apical half of the pulp canal of $\overline{4|}$.

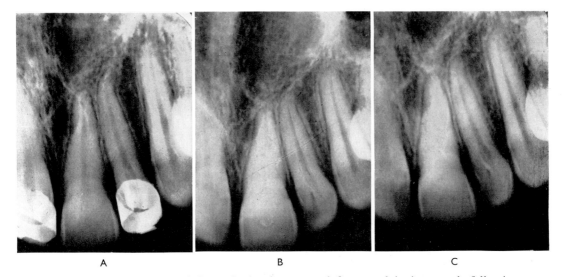

| A | B | C |

Fig. 257.—Calcification of the pulp in the upper left central incisor tooth following an injury at the age of 10 years and after orthodontic treatment for proclined upper incisors begun at the age of 11 years. **A**, Aged 13 years, February, 1954. Discoloration; diminished vitality. Radiograph: Negative. **B**, Aged 14 years, October 13, 1955. Further discoloration; diminishing response to E.C. Radiograph: Obliteration of pulp canal except apical third. **C**, Aged 15 years, August 14, 1956. Marked darkening; negative E.C. response. Radiograph: Complete obliteration of pulp canal.

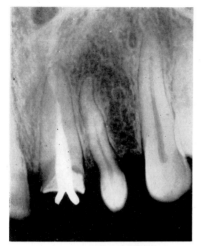

Fig. 258.—Patient, aged 31 years. Calcification of the distal half of the pulp canal. Attenuated maldeveloped tooth with irregular shaped root. Necrosis of the pulp has affected the growth of the tooth. Fell off a roundabout on to face at age of 9 years.

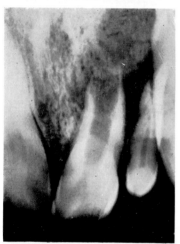

Fig. 259.—Patient, aged 27 years. Open apex hæmatoma. Blow on face at 7 years of age. Was unaware of condition, except that the lateral incisor "never grew bigger". Developed a large painful swelling after an attack of inflammation of the gums.

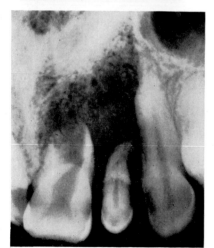

Fig. 260.—Another view of *Fig.* 259, showing the stunted growth of the lateral incisor, due to interference with the blood-supply.

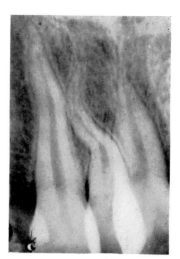

Fig. 261.—Patient, aged 19 years. 2|. Dilacerated root. Received a blow on the mouth by a cricket bat at the age of 10 years.

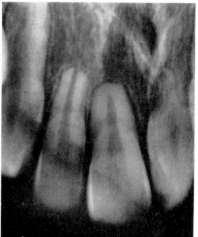

Fig. 262.—Patient, aged 13 years. Apical resorption of 21|. Blunting of roots 21|. Socket contracted down to enclose the shortened root. Fell on face the previous year. The two right upper incisors were loose for three months. There is a uniform loss of dentine and cementum, leaving a smooth convex or flattened surface at the end of the resorbed root.

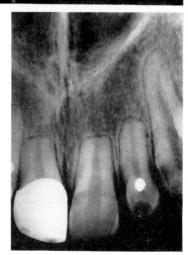

Fig. 263.—Patient, aged 18 years. Apical resorption of 1|12. Trapeze artist. No actual injury, but his "act" included biting a metal bar during a swinging turn. The lamina dura at the apices are neither thickened nor broken.

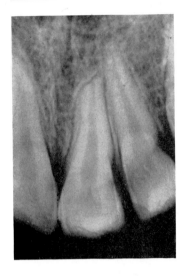

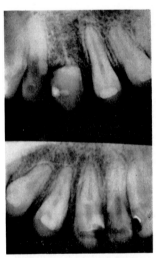

Fig. 264.—Patient, aged 13 years. Apical resorption of |1. History of trauma 12 months previously. New formation of apical socket without any cortical sclerosis.

Fig. 265.—Patient, aged 13 years. Root completely resorbed. No history of blow or local trauma. |3 is inside the bite. Histological report, after extraction of crown, states: "Repair tissue in the pulp chamber is possibly a reaction to trauma." Resorption of root probably due to occlusal trauma.

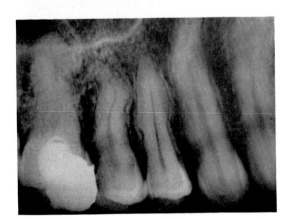

Fig. 266.—Hypercementosis of 4| with adaptation of the lamina dura without obliteration of the periodontal membrane shadow.

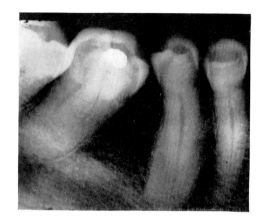

Fig. 267.—Hypercementosis of $\overline{5|}$. Large overgrowth of the cementum around the distal part of the root of $\overline{5|}$ within the socket. The appearance of the apex root is suggestive of resorption of the apex before the laying down of the new cementum.

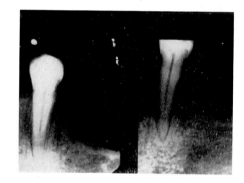

Fig. 268.—Apical bone deposition. The new bone is a cluster formation around the apical socket.

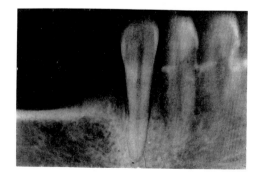

Fig. 269.—$\overline{3|}$. Another example of bone cluster formation.

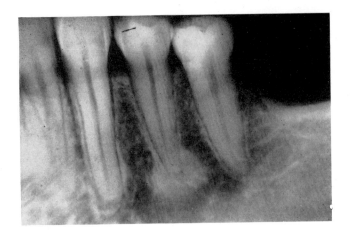

Fig. 270.—Male, aged 31 years. Spherical homogeneous sclerotic bone formed around the apex of $\overline{|4}$ outside the socket. History of a blow in this area about eighteen months previously.

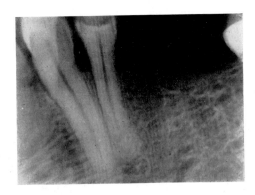

Fig. 271.—Female, aged 30 years. Ankylosis of apex with obliteration of the periodontal membrane shadow. Hit with golf club a year previously.

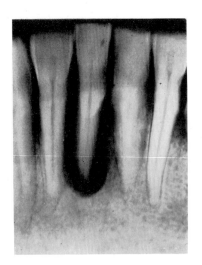

Fig. 272.—Male, aged 21 years. $\overline{1|}$. History of blow five months before. Centrifugal spread of bone destruction to the alveolar margin. Resorption of tip of apex.

Dental Caries

DENTAL caries is a widely prevalent, progressive, degenerative process of the teeth, of bacterial origin.

The presence of caries is a potential danger to the general well-being of the patient. It is an important cause of loss of the teeth, and may interfere considerably with mastication, digestion, and with the occlusion of the permanent teeth.

The infection begins at the enamel surface and, having involved the pulp, may spread along the pulp canal into the bony alveolus of the maxilla or mandible and initiate a serious systemic disturbance.

The condition is seen both in the deciduous and permanent dentitions. The teeth of late childhood and adolescence are more susceptible than those of the adult, and the rapidity of decay is greater in the younger person. The acute form of dental caries is found mostly in children and adolescents; the deciduous molars and permanent first molars are most commonly affected. When carious lesions are located in the lower incisor teeth and in the cervical areas of other teeth this is often indicative of a high degree of carious activity.

Chronic caries is a gradual disintegration of the tooth substance, commonly found in the older person where changes in the pulp proceed slowly.

It is the calcified structures of the crown of the tooth, the enamel and dentine, which are first involved, but the lesions vary in their location and form. The poorly calcified tooth may be more vulnerable than the normal crown.

The extent of involvement and the rapidity of its penetration and destruction are related to the diet, to the general standard of oral hygiene, and to the chemical composition of enamel. There are also a number of other aetiological factors of variable importance.

An accepted classification of caries is based upon:—

1. Primary Caries occurring in anatomical pits and fissures and on smooth-surface areas of stagnation.

2. Secondary Caries originating in the margins of pre-existing restorations.

3. Arrested Caries.

1. Primary Caries, starting on the surface of the crown, may be subdivided into:—

a. Occlusal Caries, which begins in anatomical pits and fissures, the latter extending into adjacent buccal and lingual surfaces. The lesion penetrates into dentine, where more rapid lateral extension undermines the overlying enamel and gives rise to its gradual or sudden collapse, with the formation of a large and clinically obvious cavity.

b. Cervical Caries most commonly affects the buccal and lingual aspects of the tooth. The lesion begins, due to stagnation, upon smooth surfaces and, in its early stages, tends generally to be shallow. Later in its development, undermining of the enamel takes place.

In both these types of caries, radiography is of limited value, since only well-developed lesions can be detected, and these are usually clinically obvious when

9

located on accessible surfaces. Occasionally, however, the advanced fissure cavity, unaccompanied by obvious enamel break-down, and the deep subgingival cavity previously unsuspected, may first be detected by radiography.

c. Interproximal Caries, originating at the contact point or in the "area of close-approach", is another important type of smooth surface caries. The initial enamel lesion is small in extent, and extensive undermining of lateral and occlusal enamel occurs.

With the destruction of the contact point, food impaction may give rise to partial destruction of the interdental gingival papilla. This, in turn, may cause radiographically visible resorption of the interdental alveolar crest.

It is in this field of the interproximal lesion that radiography plays its most important role in caries detection. The earliest lesion is inaccessible to clinical examination, but is clearly visible, from a very early stage, by use of the bite-wing technique.

2. Secondary Caries is a term commonly used to denote the recurrence of caries at the margin of an existing restoration. It may occur extensively and may ultimately involve the pulp. It can be rapid but, more commonly, it is slow in development.

Although the initial marginal failure may be clinically detectable, radiographic examination may assist in demonstrating an inaccessible lesion and also in determining the extent of carious development.

It should be noted that the carious process may also involve any tooth or fragment of tooth which is exposed to stagnation in the oral environment. Fractured surfaces, exposed root surfaces and root fragments, and partially erupted teeth may all be involved. In many of these radiography may expose the unsuspected lesion or it may determine the extent of a known cavity and its relation to the pulp.

3. Arrested Caries may occur in areas where an established lesion becomes, for one of several reasons, self-cleansing. This may arise when extensive break-down of enamel in a shallow cavity opens the cavity to the abrading effect of normal mastication, as sometimes happens in the deciduous dentition and, less frequently, in adult life.

The carious surface is dark brown, hard, and eburnated, and the progress of the lesion may be virtually arrested, or only very slowly progressive. Extraction of an adjacent tooth may be the cause of arrest of an early enamel lesion of the interproximal type.

By their nature, these forms are easily visible and radiology can contribute little in their elucidation.

Radiographic Examination of Dental Caries.—The angulation employed in intra-oral radiography to determine the existence of periapical disease produces a distorted picture of the crown of the tooth. This can be overcome to a great extent by the bite-wing technique.

Bite-wing radiography is the only method which will accurately depict pulpal conditions and marginal alveolar lesions. It should be employed to follow up the stages and degrees of penetration of caries through the enamel.

The penetration may be shown to be limited to a small defect of the enamel and will give an indication of the presence of a lesion in the underlying dentine. The clinical extent of the dentinal involvement is always found to exceed the area of detectable radiolucency. Bearing this in mind, the relation of the cavity to the pulp and the reaction of the pulp to encroachment of the caries may be determined.

In those patients where the forward inclination of the front teeth in the upper and lower jaws is exaggerated, it is recommended that the maxillary and mandibular teeth be radiographed separately.

The onset of caries is insidious and the dental care of the child should start as early as possible in its life. It would seem advisable to carry out routine radiographic examination of the teeth in children from about 4 years of age, since early detection of caries of deciduous teeth is of first importance.

In most cases, radiographic examination should be performed every six months, and in adults an annual bite-wing check should prove an adequate control, except in patients with severe caries incidence.

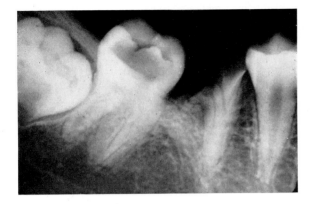

Fig. 273.—Extensive occlusal caries of a permanent lower right second molar tooth, with a retained mesial root of the first molar tooth in situ.

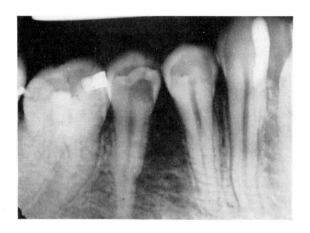

Fig. 274.—Coronal caries in the right lower second premolar tooth, involving the pulp. The lesion has spread from an initial occlusal focus.

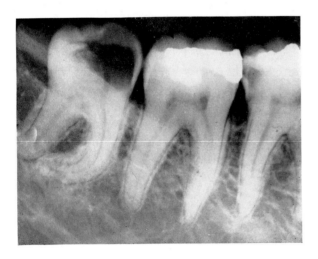

Fig. 275.—Complete coronal involvement of the lower right third molar, of occlusal origin. There is a cavity of moderate severity in the distal aspect of the first molar tooth.

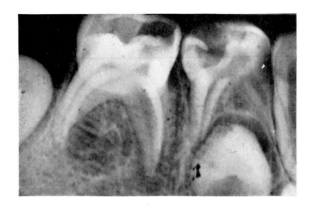

Fig. 276.—Extensive occlusal caries of the deciduous right mandibular molars.

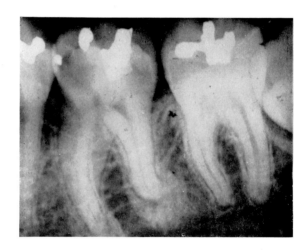

Fig. 277.—Large mesial and distal molar cavities arising from carious involvement of occlusal fissures. There is condensing osteitis around the apex of the distal root of the $\overline{6}$.

Fig. 278.—Moderate carious involvement of interstitial incisor surfaces of $\underline{12}$. The periapical lesion in this case was the result of a blow suffered one year previously.

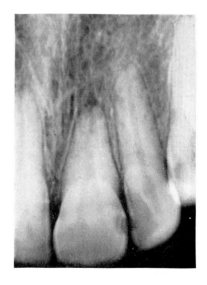

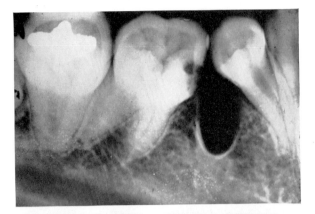

Fig. 279.—Lower permanent first right molar tooth showing a mesial cavity at point of contact with an instanding premolar tooth now extracted.

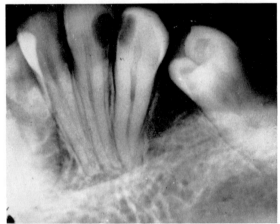

Fig. 280.—Extensive cavities in lower left incisor and canine teeth, probably involving the pulp of the former.

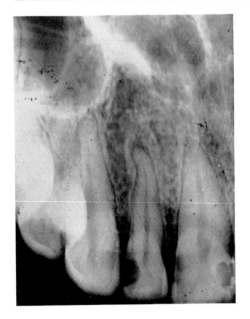

Fig. 281.—Necrosis of the lateral incisor pulp with early periapical granuloma. This is probably due to an unlined silicate filling, since the cavity is sharp in outline and does not appear to have invaded the pulp chamber.

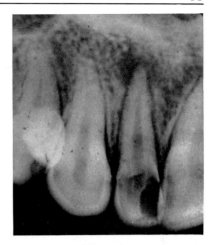

Fig. 282.—Extensive coronal destruction of the upper right lateral incisor, invading the pulp chamber with necrosis of the pulp and a periapical granuloma.

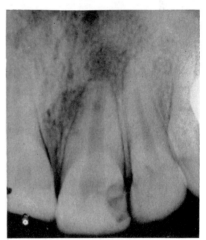

Fig. 283.—An extensive carious lesion which, with operative interference, involved the pulp of the upper left central incisor before completion of its apex. This has resulted in chronic periapical infection.

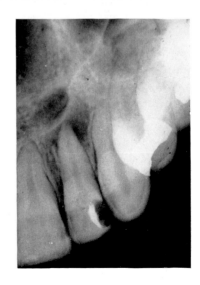

Fig. 284.—Necrosis of the maxillary lateral incisor pulp under a silicate filling lined with zinc oxyphosphate. A globular periapical granuloma has resulted.

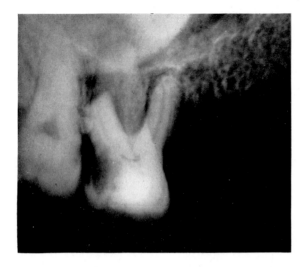

Fig. 285.—A functionless upper left first molar tooth with extensive distal cavity, necrosis of the pulp, apical resorption, and periapical infection.

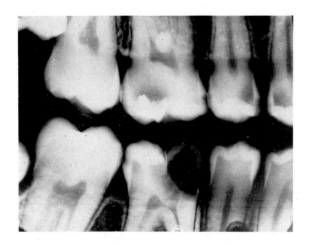

Fig. 286.—Varying degrees of interstitial and occlusal caries, from simple enamel involvement to virtually complete coronal destruction.

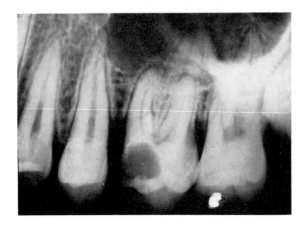

Fig. 287.—Carious exposure of the upper first molar pulp in which only a mild degree of apical periodontitis is seen against the shadow of the antrum.

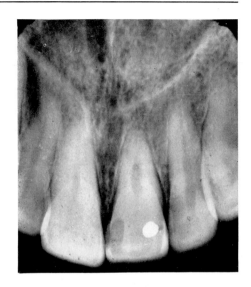

Fig. 288.—Partial obliteration of the pulp canal of the |1 due to trauma, and unconnected with the mesial and distal fillings. The apparent apical resorption may be true, but may also be due to slight retroclination of the tooth.

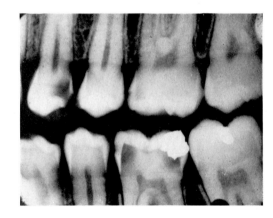

Fig. 289.—The |4 shows an extensive carious cavity on its distal aspect. The |5 shows an early lesion confined to the enamel, with a definite dental involvement in the mesial aspect of the |6. The |6 exhibits an extensive mesial cavity, occlusal fissure caries, and secondary caries below a defective distal restoration.

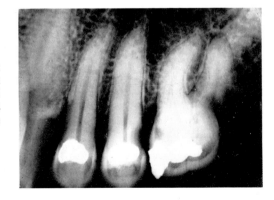

Fig. 290.—Failure of contact due to an inadequate molar restoration has resulted in food packing. Destruction of the interdental papilla and septum accompanies deep carious involvement, probably with infection of the premolar pulp.

Periapical Disease

PERIAPICAL disease embraces all lesions of an inflammatory nature, traumatic or bacterial in origin, which are located in and around the apex of a tooth or root. The pathological changes at this site may develop from within or without the tooth socket, from the tooth itself, or from the surrounding bone structure. In some cases, the infection may be blood-borne.

The changes occur in the closest proximity to the apical end of the tooth and involve all the tissues, soft and hard, situated in this limited area.

These periapical lesions are subject to progressive and retrogressive variations which may take place simultaneously in the tissues surrounding the apex of the tooth and its pedicle of nutrient vessels and nerves.

The inflammatory reaction may be acute or chronic and involve the terminal part of the pulp canal, the apical cementum and dentine, the periodontal membrane, the lamina dura of the distal end of the socket, and the cortical bone of the alveolar process. Which of these structures becomes affected, the order of attack, and sequence of destruction depend upon the cause of the lesion, the point of origin, the direction of spread of the disease, and the severity of the infection.

The reaction of the tissues to inflammation is governed by the number and virulence of the invading organisms and the resistance of the patient. Although the tendency is towards disorganization and destruction of the body tissues, arrest of the disease can occur at any stage with subsequent repair of the destroyed tissue.

Radiography is invaluable in depicting the presence of a pathological condition. In some instances it is the sole means of an early diagnosis.

Repetitive films taken under standard conditions should reveal the presence of progressive tissue resorption or the arrest of the destructive condition. Repair is shown in the deposition of new bone formation.

In the early stages of acute inflammation, before the hard structures have been involved, no definite radiographic signs are visible. As soon as abnormal shadows are seen around the apex, the lesion has passed into the sub-acute or chronic phase.

The swelling of the inflamed periodontal membrane around the apex of the tooth cannot be seen on a radiograph. The soft tissues do not cast any shadow on the film. When the engorged enlargement of the membrane persists for any length of time, the hard encompassing structures of the cementum and lamina dura become eroded, and the normal thin linear black image between the root and the socket on the radiograph will appear thickened and irregular.

The opaque structure of a root or of the bone is demonstrable on a radiograph, showing an erosion of the apical part of the tooth or a break in the continuity of the lamina dura. As the periapical disease progresses destruction or resorption of the root can be seen, and extension into the osseous support to the tooth is depicted as loss of the bone pattern with rarefaction.

Except in the case of trauma, periapical disease begins at a carious area on the crown of the tooth and sets up a pulpitis with death of the pulp. The inflammatory process travels along the pulp canal to the apical end of the root and the infection reaches the outer surface of the tooth through minute openings at the apex and then into the surrounding periodontal membrane.

The various changes which may take place in the immediate structures, extending radially from this site, are shown in the following radiographic illustrations.

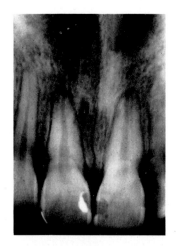

Fig. 291.—1|1. Slight thickening and irregularity of the apical periodontal membrane shadows. Both crowns show carious cavitation.

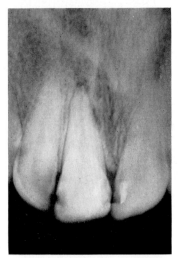

Fig. 292.—1|. Coronal caries. Thickening and irregularity of the periodontal membrane shadow at the apex and on the mesial side of the root. Signs of erosion of the distal part of the root.

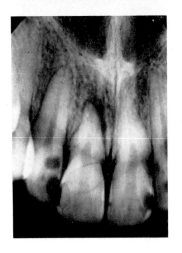

Fig. 293.—Thickening and irregularity of the apical periodontal membrane shadow with erosion of the mesial lamina dura. Localized rarefying osteitis on the mesial aspect of the root of 1|.

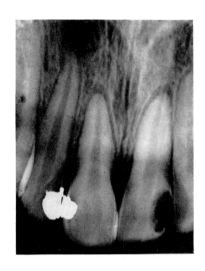

Fig. 294.—Subluxation of both upper central incisor teeth. The periodontal membrane shadows show a tapering widening but no irregularity. No erosion of the lamina dura. No signs of rarefying osteitis.

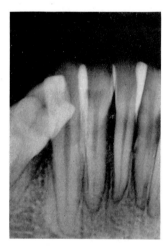

Fig. 295.—$\overline{3|}$. Localized periapical condensing osteitis around the apex.

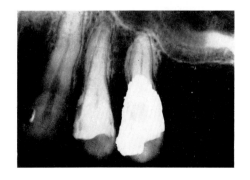

Fig. 296.—Linear condensing osteitis enveloping the socket of $\underline{|5}$ in a heavily filled tooth.

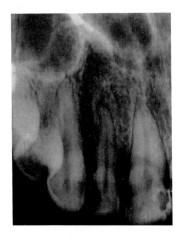

Fig. 297.—Periapical condensing osteitis in ring formation around a residual swelling of the apical periodontal membrane of 2|.

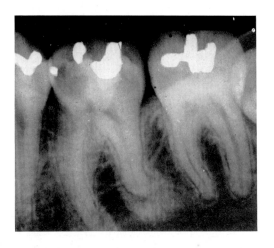

Fig. 298.—Localized homogeneous bulbous periapical condensing osteitis around the distal apex of |6̄.

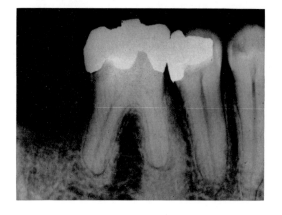

Fig. 299.—Periapical bony sclerosis enclosing the apices of 6̄|, which show limited resorption.

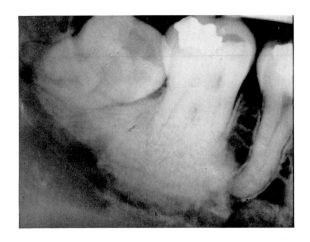

Fig. 300.—Diffused sclerosis around the roots of $\overline{87|}$. The obliteration of the periodontal membrane shadow shows the existence of ankylosis.

Fig. 301.—Extensive sclerosis around a retained root fragment.

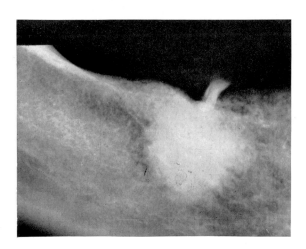

Fig. 302.—Cementosis of the distal half of $4|$ root. Excess deposition of cementum showing change of root formation within the socket. The lamina dura has adapted itself to the new formation, without the obliteration of the periodontal membrane shadow.

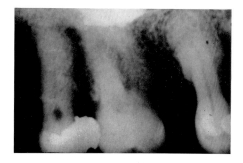

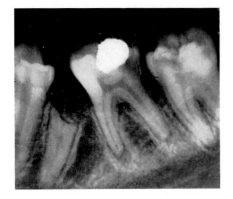

Fig. 303.—Slowly progressive resorption of the apices of $\overline{6}$ with concurrent deposition immediately outside the socket of reparative new bone.

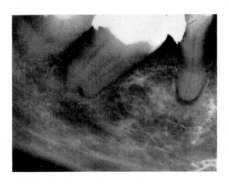

Fig. 304.—Cementosis of the distal halves of the roots of $\overline{65}|$ with concurrent reparative new bone formation.

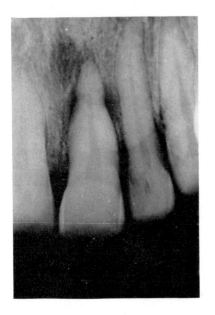

Fig. 305.—Encircling erosion of the distal half of the root of $\underline{1}$.

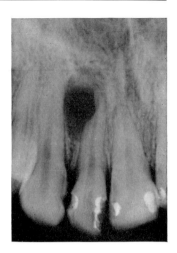

Fig. 306.—Rarefying osteitis destroying the mesial part of the apex of 2| and extending laterally to 3|.

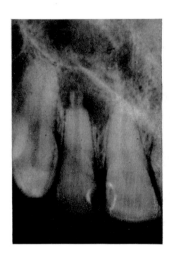

Fig. 307.—Progressive inflammatory re-sorption of the apex of 2| in an abscess cavity.

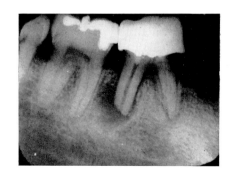

Fig. 308.—Inflammatory resorption of the distal root of 6| with the abscess tracking its way towards the alveolar margin.

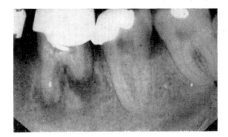

Fig. 309.—Advanced resorption of the apices of the roots of 6̄|. The inflammatory destructive process is localized to the socket areas.

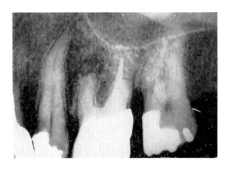

Fig. 310.—The mesial root of |6 is stunted as a result of resorption. The reconstructed distal half of the socket is of cancellous and not of sclerosed bone.

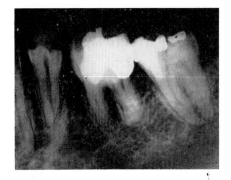

Fig. 311.—Oblique resorption of the apex of |5. The periodontal membrane shadow in this area shows no thickening or irregularity and there is an elongated sclerotic reinforcement on the distal side of the socket.

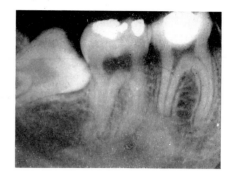

Fig. 312.—The active resorption of the apex of the distal root of 6̅| has been arrested and the destroyed bone replaced by a non-trabeculated mass of sclerosed bone.

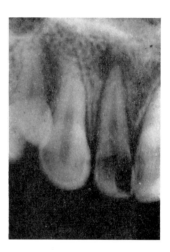

Fig. 313.—Typical appearance of a chronic apical abscess associated with 2̲|. There is a large carious cavity in the crown.

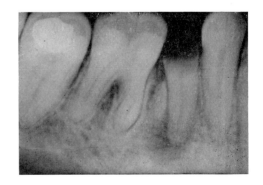

Fig. 314.—Retained root 5̅| with a periapical dento-alveolar abscess.

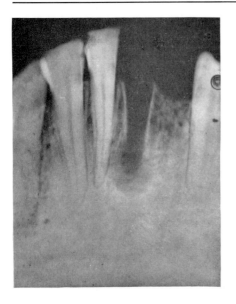

Fig. 315.—Dento-alveolar abscess. Empty socket of ⌐1 showing the destruction of the apical lamina dura and rarefying osteitis beyond the apex.

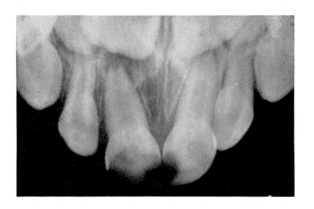

Fig. 316.—Apical abscess in connexion with A⌐.

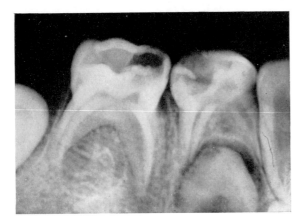

Fig. 317.—Apical abscess in connexion with E⌐.

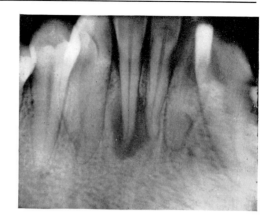

Fig. 318.—Chronic dento-alveolar abscess. Localized periapical area of rarefying osteitis with bone destruction. No erosion of the apex. Root appears to be dipping into the abscess cavity.

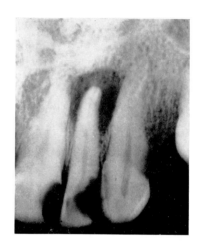

Fig. 319.—Rarefying destructive osteitis. A periapical granuloma has broken down into a dento-alveolar abscess.

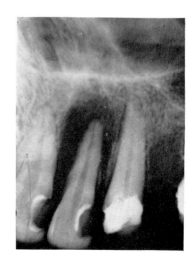

Fig. 320.—Rarefying destructive osteitis beginning as a periapical lesion; the extension of the bone destruction has been towards the alveolar margin. The bony interdental septa on both sides of the affected tooth have been destroyed. There is usually a fistulous discharge at the gingival margin in these cases.

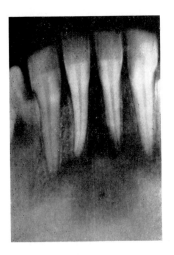

Fig. 321.—Rarefying destructive osteitis. The spread of the destructive process is lateral across to the outer wall of the socket of the neighbouring teeth.

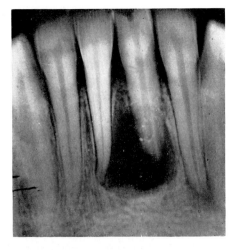

Fig. 322.—The apex of $\overline{1|}$ is gradually being eroded and resorbed while the abscess area is spreading to the $\overline{1|}$ towards the alveolar margin and beyond the apex.

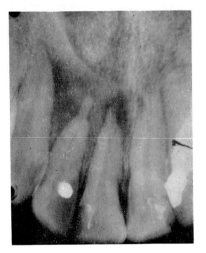

Fig. 323.—The apices of $\underline{1|}$ and $\underline{2|}$ are involved separately, each undergoing destruction and resorption. The base of the bony interdental septum acts as a partition between the two abscess cavities.

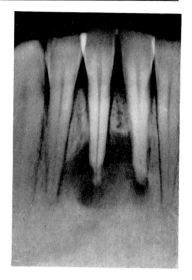

Fig. 324.—There is a large confluent abscess around the apices of 1|1 with erosion of both apices and disintegration of the intervening bony interdental septa.

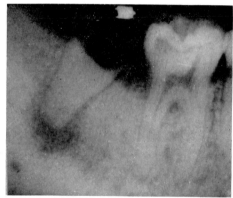

Fig. 325.—The spreading destructive osteitis from the apex of 8| has encroached upon the mental foramen and inferior dental canal.

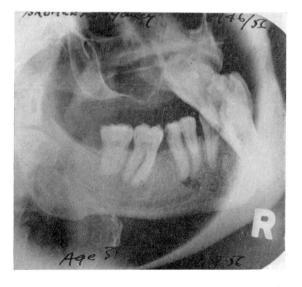

Fig. 326.—The localized dento-alveolar abscess at the apex of 5| lies adjacent to, but has not penetrated into, the mental foramen.

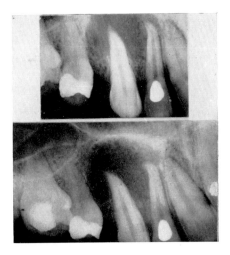

Fig. 327.—The rarefying destructive osteitis has extended centrifugally away from the apex of 43| region towards and into the floor of the maxillary antrum.

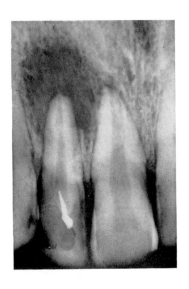

Fig. 328.—The rarefying osteitis arising from 2| is moving towards the floor of the nasal fossa.

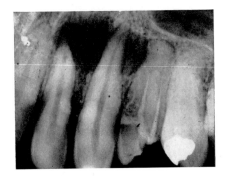

Fig. 329.—The oval-shaped black area incorporates the apices of the |234 and is a periapical abscess arising from |4. It is tracking behind the |23 on the palatal side of their apices.

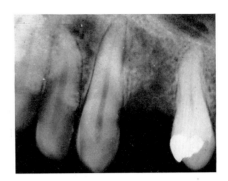

Fig. 330.—Same patient as in Fig. 329 after the extraction of |4 six weeks previously. Efficient drainage of the pus was effected and the laminæ dura of |23 show no signs of apical periodontitis.

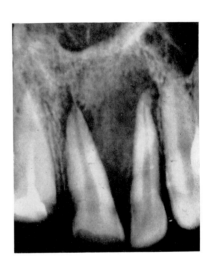

Fig. 331.—The large dento-alveolar abscess in the |12 region has produced a divarication of the roots with approximation of their crowns. At operation the abscess was contained in a fibrous sac.

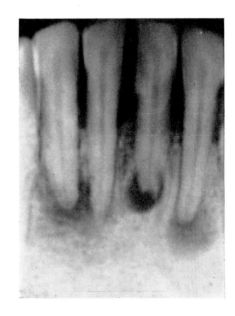

Fig. 332.—Each apex of $\overline{21|12}$ has a dento-alveolar abscess.

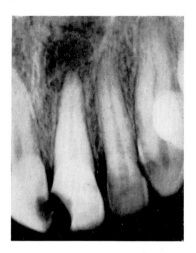

Fig. 333.—Apical granuloma. A rounded dark area is seen at the apex of the |1 continuous with the periodontal membrane shadow of the tooth, and encompassed by a limiting structure. The internal small dark spots indicate a breaking down of a central mass.

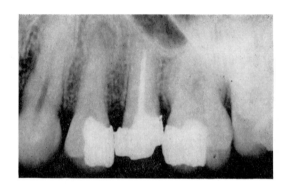

Fig. 334.—Around the apical granuloma associated with |5 a cortical circular wall has been formed. This wall is continuous with the lamina dura of the socket.

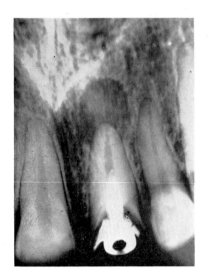

Fig. 335.—The apical granuloma in the |1 region is well defined and the various degrees of rarefaction indicate vacuolation.

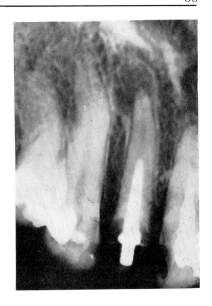

Fig. 336.—The granuloma formed at the end of the apex of 2| is a potential radicular cyst and may encroach upon the right nasal fossa.

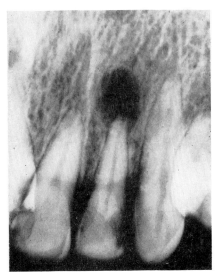

Fig. 337.—The enclosed area of the granuloma at the apex of |2 is definitely blacker as a result of its fluid contents.

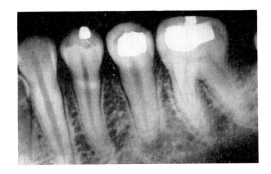

Fig. 338.—The granuloma at the apex of |5 may grow and extend downwards to the mental foramen and inferior dental canal.

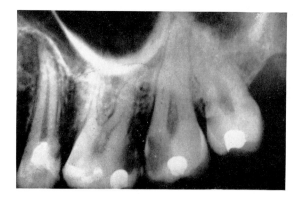

Fig. 339.—|5. Apical granuloma lying just below the floor of the left antrum.

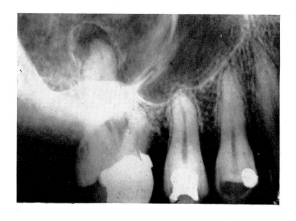

Fig. 340.—6|. Apical granuloma lying lateral to the forward loculus of the right antrum. It has not penetrated through into the loculus.

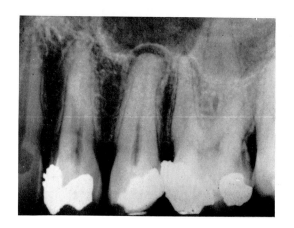

Fig. 341.—|5. Apical granuloma invaginating the floor of the left antrum.

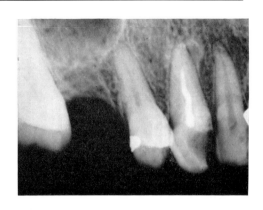

Fig. 342.—Apical granuloma lying to the mesial side of the apex of 4|.

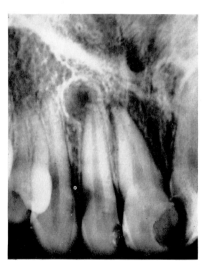

Fig. 343.—Apical granuloma lying to the lateral side of the apex of 2|.

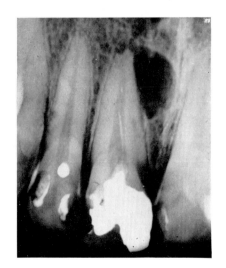

Fig. 344.—Apical granuloma lying to the mesial side of 1|. The last three examples are forerunners of the less common lateral periodontal cysts.

Marginal Periodontitis

MARGINAL periodontitis usually begins as a chronic inflammatory condition of the gums. The gingivitis may proceed to involve the underlying periodontal membrane covering the alveolar process with eventual destruction and recession of the immediate bone.

The resorption of the supporting bone of the teeth, if localized, results in "pocket" formation with increasing mobility of the tooth in its socket.

Gingivitis is found at all ages, even in childhood, and recession of the alveolar bone is often observed, especially in later life, without any apparent change in the gum margins.

No radiographic changes are seen until the marginal periodontal membrane is affected and then the first signs are irregular widening of the black periodontal shadow around the cervical margins of the teeth.

Radiographic examination reveals the subsequent destructive phases of marginal periodontal disease, demonstrating resorption of the summits of the bony interdental septa, widespread recession of the alveolar bone, and attendant root changes of erosion and resorption.

At the same time the periodontologist acknowledges the invaluable information which he is able to receive by repetitive radiographic observation during the treatment of a patient suffering from marginal periodontitis. The demonstration of the arrest of bone destruction is of great importance in the assessment of the local reaction to repair. The mere absence of bone regeneration is not evidence of unsuccessful treatment.

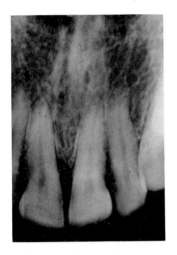

Fig. 345.—Destruction of the summit of the bony interdental septum between the upper central teeth, due to direct injury.

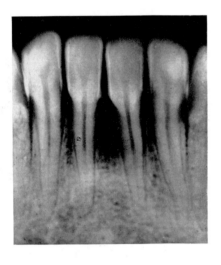

Fig. 346.—Resorption of the apex of the bony interdental septum between the lower central incisors, with thickening of the cervical marginal periodontal membrane.

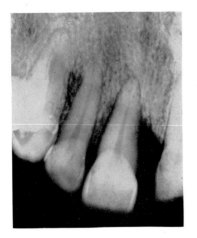

Fig. 347.—Resorption of the bony interdental septum between the upper central teeth. The socket walls of 1| have also been destroyed, all due to the spread of local gingivitis to the underlying periodontium.

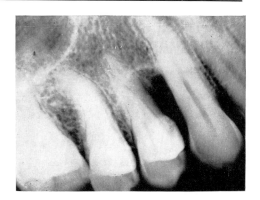

Fig. 348.—The alveolar bone destruction is confined to 43|, denuding their roots of the socket wall. The intervening supporting interdental bony septum also has been resorbed.

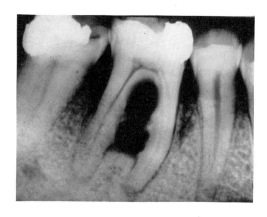

Fig. 349.—Localized marginal periodontitis with destruction of the inter-radicular bony septum 6̄|.

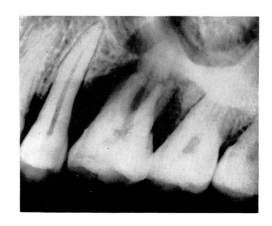

Fig. 350.—Progressive marginal periodontitis with resorption of the alveolar bone around |6 extending to the |5 and |7 on either side.

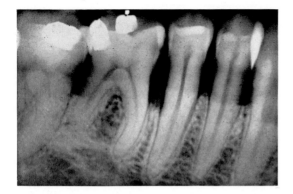

Fig. 351.—The marginal perio-
dontitis involves the $\overline{654|}$. The
"horizontal" alveolar resorption produces shallow pocket formation.

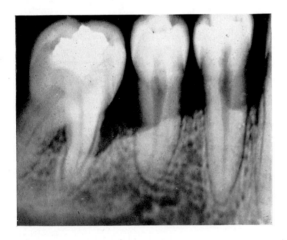

Fig. 352.—The recession of the
alveolar bone has caused deep pocket-
ing between $\overline{5|}$ and $\overline{6|}$. This is de-
scribed as "vertical" periodontitis.

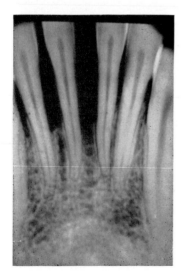

Fig. 353.—Localized marginal periodon-
titis is confined to the $\overline{21|12}$ region with
resorption of the marginal bone.

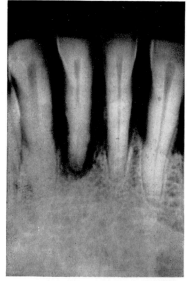

Fig. 354.—The progressive "horizontal" periodontitis in the 21|12 region has produced almost total loss of bony support.

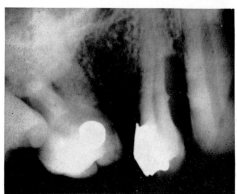

Fig. 355.—The marginal periodontitis is eroding the mesial aspect of the root of 4|.

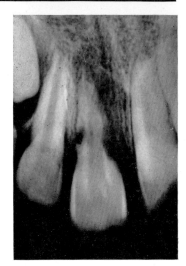

Fig. 356.—There is an encircling resorption of the cervical region of the 1|. The rarefying osteitis is involving the mesial bony inter-dental septum with the formation of a parodontal-periapical abscess.

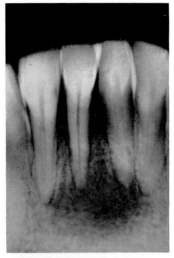

Fig. 357.—Relatively mild marginal periodontitis producing resorption of the bony
interdental septum in the $\overline{21|1}$ region. A
secondary periapical abscess has developed.

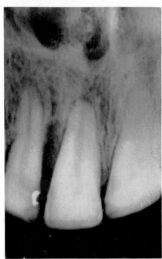

Fig. 358.—The gingival inflammation is
localized to the area between the upper
right and lateral incisor teeth. A rarefying
"canalized" area is tracking up to the apical
region.

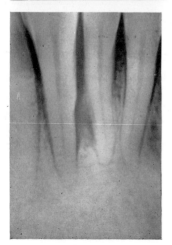

Fig. 359.—Formation of a small parodontal
abscess between the lower right central and
lateral incisor teeth.

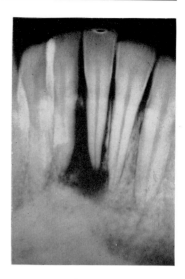

Fig. 360.—Parodontal abscess between the lower right central and lateral incisors, extending from the alveolar margin to the apical region and completely destroying the bony interdental septa.

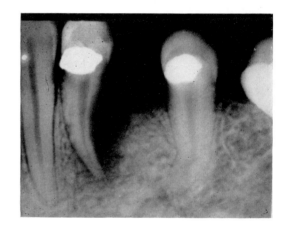

Fig. 361.—Large parodontal abscess lateral to the ⌐4 eroding the root and destroying the alveolar bone.

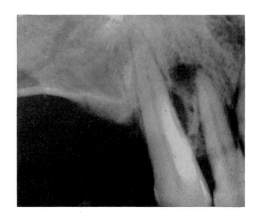

Fig. 362.—Confined parodontal abscess on the mesial aspect of 3|. There is no recession of the apex of the bony interdental septum. There is a periapical abscess associated with 2|.

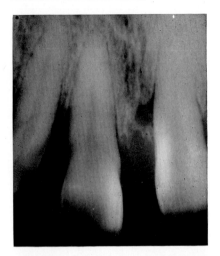

Fig. 363.—Localized parodontal abscess mesial to |1.

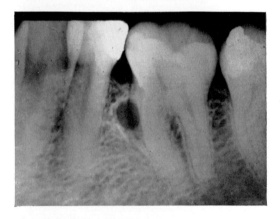

Fig. 364.—Parodontal abscess mesial to |6 surrounded by a well circumscribed wall.

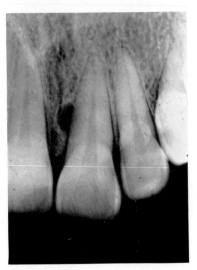

Fig. 365.—Well contained parodontal abscess mesial to |1.

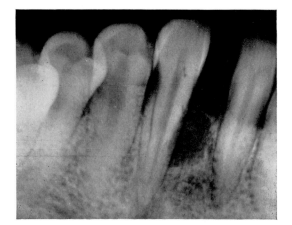

Fig. 366.—Parodontal abscess mesial to $\overline{3|}$ slowly advancing to the $\overline{2|}$.

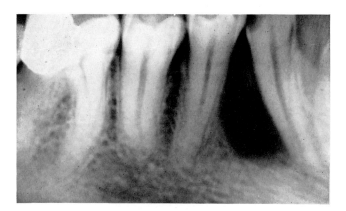

Fig. 367.—Large parodontal abscess completely destroying the bony interdental septum between $\overline{3|}$ and $\overline{4|}$.

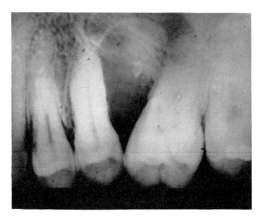

A

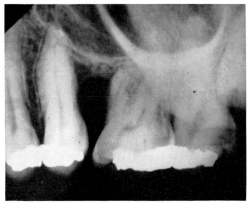

B

Fig. 368.—A, Parodontal abscess between $|\underline{5}$ and $|\underline{6}$. B, Same case twelve months after treatment, showing bone regeneration.

Internal Root Resorption. Idiopathic Resorption of the Root

INTERNAL root resorption is an obscure condition of unknown aetiology. Whereas external root resorption is due to chronic periapical infection, the idiopathic resorption of the pulp wall is now claimed to be neoplastic in origin.

The resorption may start either from within the pulp or in the periodontal membrane in the tooth socket. The changes which take place result in the gradual resorption of the pulp chamber or canal. Eventually the dentine is resorbed and a communication often effected between the pulp and the periodontal membrane. At the same time metaplastic changes take place, with the transformation of local dental tissue into osseous tissue.

Internal root resorption has been observed in patients between the ages of 9 and 64 years and has no special preference for either sex. The condition is generally confined to a single tooth, but more than one tooth may be involved in the same patient. It occurs in both unerupted and erupted teeth, in the crown or root alone, or in both simultaneously.

Radiographically, the lesion may first be identified as an enlargement or dilatation of the pulp canal, localized or elongated. Later, it presents a circular or punched-out radiolucent black area situated in the crown or in the cervical region of the tooth. There may be an external perforation through the wall of the tooth, and sometimes there is a complete separation of the crown from the root, simulating a fracture.

In some cases the resorption appears to begin at the periphery of a tooth, often at the neck. It tends to spread inwards into the pulp cavity and may be mistaken for cervical caries.

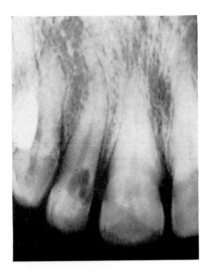

Fig. 369.—The irregular black area on the mesial half of the cervical region of the 2| appears to originate from the periphery. There is a communication between the outer surface of the tooth and the pulp canal.

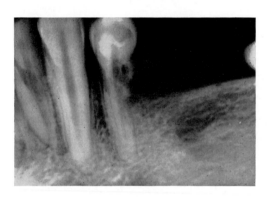

Fig. 370.—The lesion is localized to the outer surface of the distal area of the root of the |4̄ below the neck of the tooth. In addition to the destruction of the root there appears to be a metaplastic osseous deposit in this area.

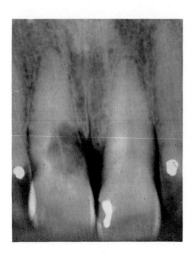

Fig. 371.—The internal root resorption in the 1| has perforated the external wall of the tooth and is extending into the crown. The pulp canal in the distal half of the root is almost obliterated.

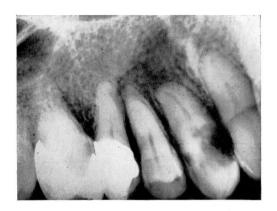

Fig. 372.—The internal root resorption has involved the proximal half of the tooth and its proximal outer wall. May be mistaken for cervical caries.

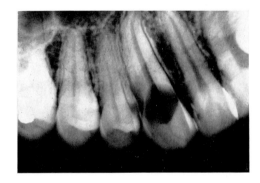

Fig. 373.—The pulp canal of 3| shows no marked change in its whole length. The lesion is identified as a circular punched-out area in the cervical region. No actual perforation can be seen.

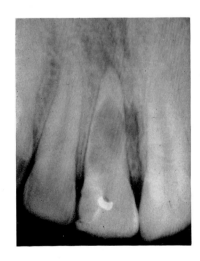

Fig. 374.—The ovoid rarefied area involves the proximal two-thirds of the root of 1|, and has perforated the outer surface with local parodontal osteitis on its mesial aspect. Note the periapical lesion.

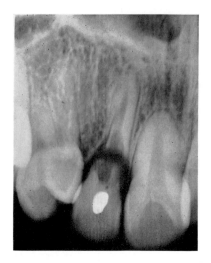

Fig. 375.—The proximal half of the pulp canal in the 2| shows an elongated dilatation. The root resorption has produced a transverse fracture of the tooth in this region.

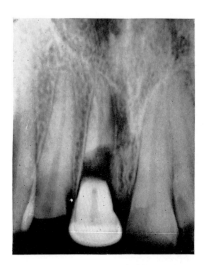

Fig. 376.—Fracture of 1| due to the resorption of the root in its middle third. Osseous metaplastic changes are seen in the punched-out radiolucent area.

Osteitis and Osteomyelitis

PERIAPICAL disease and marginal periodontitis may develop insidiously into a periapical and parodontal osteitis. The inflammation of the bone may remain localized or become more extensive in both jaws. If unchecked, the destructive process could penetrate to the nasal fossa or antrum, encroach upon the mental foramen or inferior dental canal, or extend into the floor of the mouth, or to the outer surface of the face.

The main distinction between osteitis and osteomyelitis lies in the area of the bone involved, together with toxic symptoms exhibited by the patient.

The acute stage of osteomyelitis usually declares itself as a purulent subperiosteal condition, and in the absence of bone destruction, presents no definite radiographic signs. The earliest radiographic changes are rarely seen in under seven days in acute osteomyelitis, but thereafter they follow a well recognized sequence.

The spread of the dental infection into the immediate surrounding bone produces a rarefaction in the osseous tissue, with breaking down of the bone structure and the formation of a chronic alveolar abscess. This is known as *diffuse rarefying osteitis*.

The radiograph presents a black, irregular, diffuse area, void of any definite outline and merging into the surrounding bone without any demarcation. This could be the starting point of a spreading osteomyelitis. On the other hand, there may be a local bone reaction with deposition of new bone, thus acting as a barrier to further bone destruction. This is known as *condensing osteitis*.

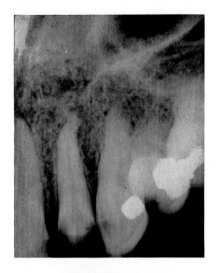

Fig. 377.—The radiolucent area around and beyond the periapical region of the |2 is due to inflammatory decalcification of the bone.

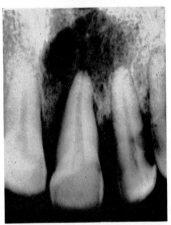

Fig. 378.—The chronic rarefying osteitis spreading from the |1 is darker on account of bone disintegration. The bone spaces are filled with chronic inflammatory granulation tissue.

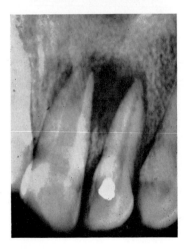

Fig. 379.—The numerous defined "black holes" are produced by the breaking down of the trabeculæ around the medullary spaces. The spaces contain pus.

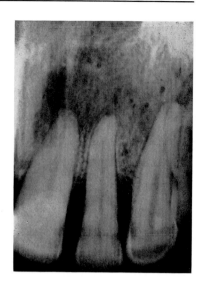

Fig. 380.—|1̲2̲. The rarefying osteitis is widespread, extending upwards to the nasal fossa. The "black holes" are abundant.

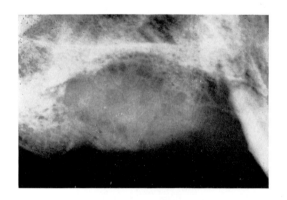

Fig. 381.—The confluent medullary spaces have increased in number and diameter. The main rarefying area has lost much of its calcification.

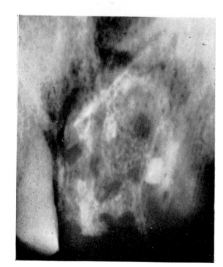

Fig. 382.—The internal circular areas of bone disintegration are enlarged. Small areas of bone are becoming isolated with eventual sequestrum formation.

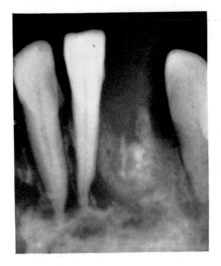

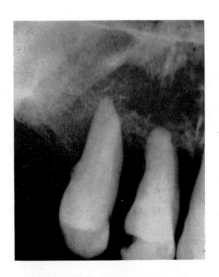

Fig. 383.—Spreading destructive osteitis with isolation of dead or dying areas of bone.

Fig. 384.—Rarefying destructive osteitis in 543| region with much loss of bone. This condition has spread by perforation of an infected right antrum.

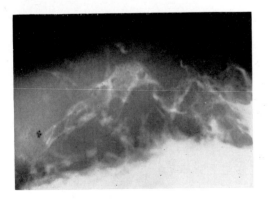

Fig. 385.—Advanced local destructive osteitis with sequestrum formation.

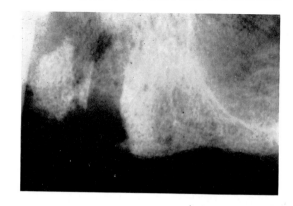

Fig. 386.—Sequestrum in |34 region following upon tooth extraction associated with a suppurative alveolar condition.

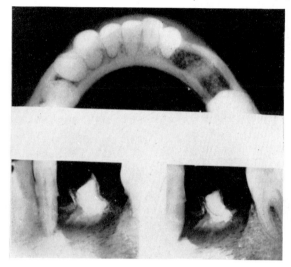

Fig. 387.—Bony sequestrum in |345 region carrying root in socket.

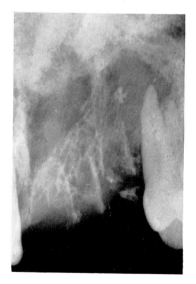

Fig. 388.—Large sequestrum embodying socket of |345 region.

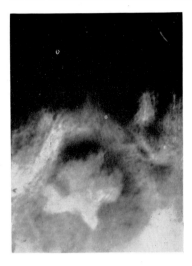

Fig. 389.—Irregular sequestrum lying in abscess area in $\overline{|345}$ region. It is important to provide active drainage of the pus in such cases.

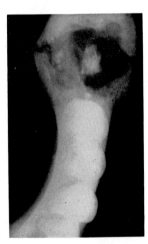

Fig. 390.—Occlusal view of $\overline{|67}$ region showing a sequestrum in a large abscess cavity. Pathological fracture of the mandible transversely due to failure of effective drainage of the pus.

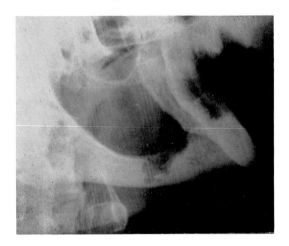

Fig. 391.—Root fragment and sequestrum in area of destructive osteitis in large abscess cavity. The bone destruction is proceeding towards the lower border.

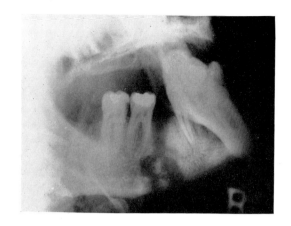

Fig. 392.—The lower right second premolar tooth has been extracted, but bone necrosis has proceeded to and through the inferior border of the mandible, leaving sequestra in its wake.

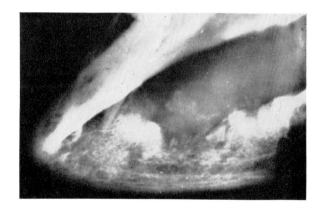

Fig. 393.—Sequestrum in $\overline{|56}$ region.

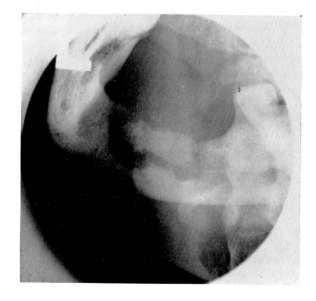

Fig. 394.—Unusually large sequestrum in the lower left mandible.

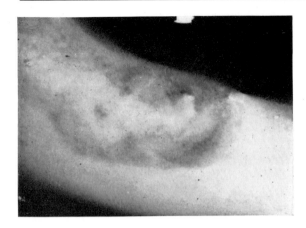

Fig. 395.—The composite sequestrum is lying in an abscess trough which is surrounded by an outer wall of condensing osteitis.

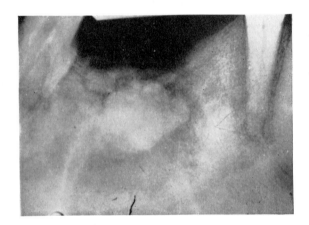

Fig. 396.—With effective drainage and increasing severance of the blood-supply, the sequestrum rises to the alveolar margin like a buoy on a mooring rope.

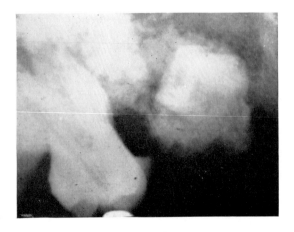

Fig. 397.—Sequestrum in the 76| region has reached the oral cavity and is in a process of exfoliation.

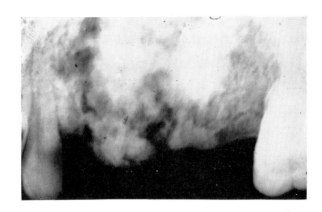

Fig. 398.—Osteomyelitis following upon traumatic osteitis in the |345 region after surgical attempt to remove an unerupted left upper canine.

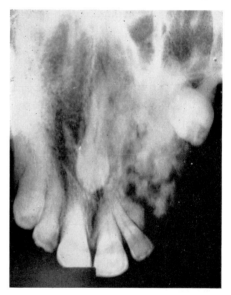

Fig. 399.—Occlusal view of *Fig.* 398 showing new bone regeneration as well as bone destruction.

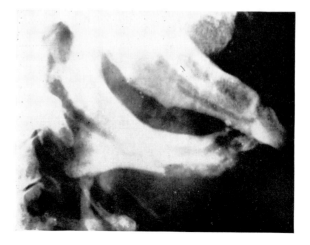

Fig. 400.—Osteomyelitis involving the mesial half of the right mandible.

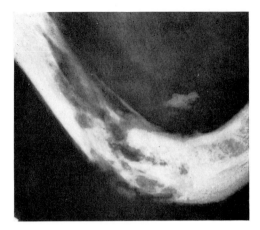

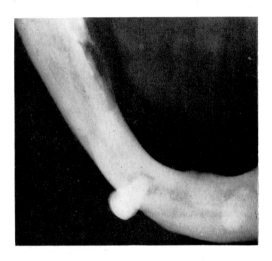

Fig. 401.—Occlusal view of *Fig.* 400. The destructive process is seen to be more widespread, and has thrown off a sequestrum into the soft tissues of the floor of the mouth.

Fig. 402.—The osteomyelitis is confined to the lingual aspect of the mandible and has penetrated into the floor of the mouth.

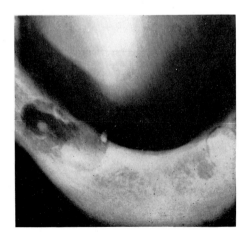

Fig. 403.—The osteomyelitis is involving the mandible in the $\overline{543|}$ region almost completely across from inner to outer walls. The area contains retained roots and sequestra.

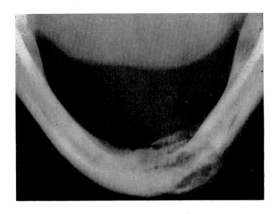

Fig. 404.—Osteomyelitis involving $\overline{|1-4}$ and extending from the inner to the outer wall.

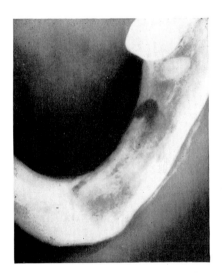

Fig. 405.—Osteomyelitis $\overline{|1-6}$. On the outer surface of the mandible is seen a thin white shadow of periostitic reaction.

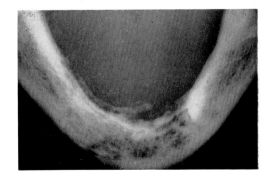

Fig. 406.—Osteomyelitis $\overline{|1-4}$ extending across the middle line to the $\overline{5|}$ region. Periostitic reaction is seen on the inner border of the mandible on the right side.

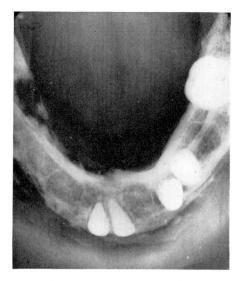

Fig. 407.—Extensive osteomyelitis from $\overline{6\text{-}|\text{-}6}$ region, with progressive destruction of the bone.

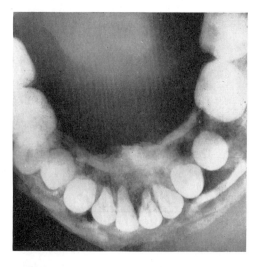

Fig. 408.—Concurrent with the destruction of the bone resulting from the osteomyelitis of $\overline{6\text{-}|\text{-}6}$, there is much periostitic reaction.

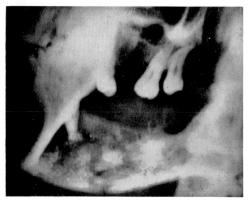

Fig. 409.—Osteomyelitis in the $\overline{|1\text{—}7}$ region with sequestrum formation and pathological fracture.

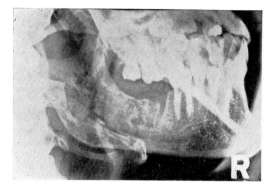

Fig. 410.—Patient, aged 25 years. Osteomyelitis of the mandible extending up the ramus to the submandibular notch. This radiograph was taken three weeks after extraction of an infected 7|. Multiple isolated areas of rarefaction with signs of sequestration.

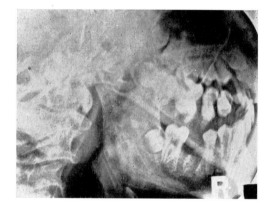

Fig. 411.—Patient, aged 13 years. Osteomyelitis of the right ramus with punctate decalcification of the bone. Painless swelling over the mandible and ramus developed insidiously after extraction of 6| six months previously.

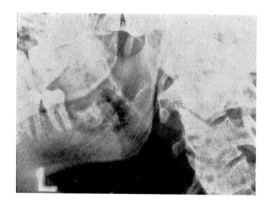

Fig. 412.—Patient, aged 39 years. Osteomyelitis in the |8 region extending upwards to the lingula of the ramus. Impacted |8 extracted five weeks previously. Well-marked sequestrum lying in |8 region.

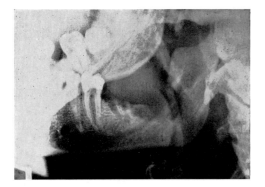

Fig. 413.—Same patient as *Fig.* 412 three months later, showing bone regeneration.

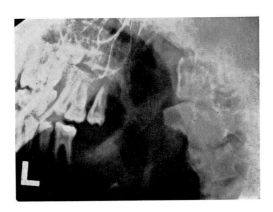

Fig. 414.—Large rarefied area of osteo-myelitis involving the whole of the coronoid process.

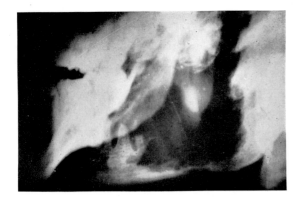

Fig. 415.—Large cavity in the mandible extending from $\overline{6}$ region up the ramus. Massive sequestrum removed three weeks previously.

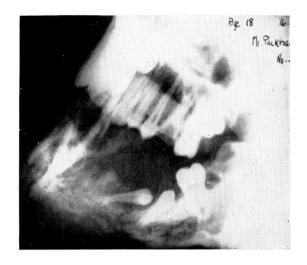

Fig. 416.—Osteomyelitis in $\overline{1-5}$ region resulting from an attempt to remove unerupted $\overline{45}$.

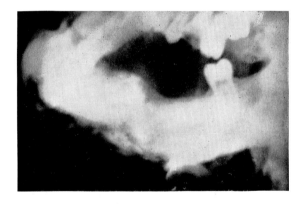

Fig. 417.—Same patient three weeks later. Widespread active osteomyelitis. $\overline{45}$ have been extracted.

Fig. 418.—Same patient one year later. Bone regeneration.

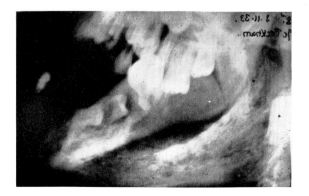

Fractures of the Teeth

INJURIES to the teeth are due, in the main, to direct blows. The anterior teeth, especially those in the maxilla, are more frequently involved.

A pathological fracture of the crown of a tooth can occur in coronal caries, in a root-filled tooth, and in root metaplasia.

An injury to a tooth may result in:—

1. Displacement of the tooth in its socket.
2. Fracture of the crown or root, or both.
3. Fracture-dislocation of the tooth.
4. Fracture of the tooth and supporting bone structure.
5. Apical hæmatoma, death of the pulp, and open apex concurrent with the fractured tooth.
6. Fracture of the tooth with an apical abscess.
7. Calcification and obliteration of the pulp canal following a fracture.
8. Dilaceration of the root after healing of the fracture.

Any form of trauma to a tooth should be followed by a radiographic examination because of a possible root fracture and involvement of the pulp chamber. This is the only way to show the position of fractured tooth fragments.

In partial dislocation, the tooth may be reduced and success could follow fixation. A tooth totally dislocated from its socket may be replanted, but usually it has to be extracted.

A *fractured crown* may show:—

1. A fissure or crack without separation of fragments.
2. A chip off the edge with involvement of the dentine, but no exposure of the pulp.
3. A transverse fracture line.
4. A vertical fracture line.
5. An oblique fracture line.
6. A comminution.
7. An extension into root.

A fractured root may be:—

1. Transverse.
2. Vertical.
3. Oblique.

A fracture of the root may occur anywhere along its length, or extend from a fractured crown. It could be associated with a break in the alveolar process.

If the root remains firm in its socket, it may retain its vitality and heal. Usually the tooth loses its vitality after a fracture.

An appreciable amount of separation between the root fragments may take place after a fracture. Separation is minimal with an oblique break of the root.

Fractured roots heal in a similar way to a bone fracture. The nearer the fracture is to the apex of the root, the more likely is it to unite. It may take three to six months for a fractured root to form a sound union.

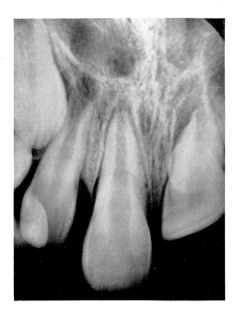

Fig. 419.—Dislocation of the teeth. 1|1. The patient reported that he had received a blow on his mouth. The left upper central is dislodged in its socket and the thickening of the apical periodontal membrane shadow of the upper right central is due to the loosening of the tooth in its socket.

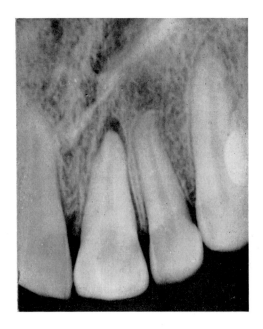

Fig. 420.—|1. Subluxation of the upper left central incisor in its socket.

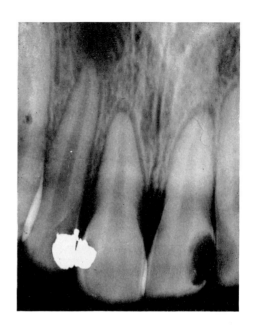

Fig. 421.—1|1. Subluxation of both upper central incisor teeth. The periodontal membrane shadows show a tapering widening but no irregularity. There is erosion of the lamina dura, and no signs of rarefying osteitis.

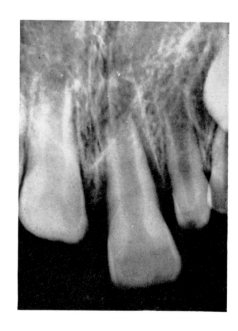

Fig. 422.—1|. The upper left central incisor tooth is grossly displaced downwards.

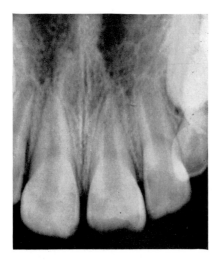

Fig. 423.—Coronal fracture. Chip fracture of the incisive edge of the crown of |1.

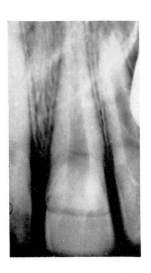

Fig. 424.—Coronal fracture. The crown of |1 is fractured by a buccopalatal oblique cleavage. The overlapping limiting edges of the crown present two separate transverse fracture lines.

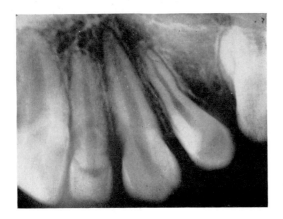

Fig. 425.—Coronal fracture. The crown of |2 shows a transverse fracture. The proximal coronal fragment is loosely connected to the root.

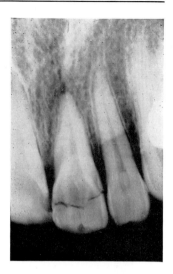

Fig. 426.—Coronal fracture. There is a transverse fracture of the crown of |1 as well as a chip fracture at the incisive edge.

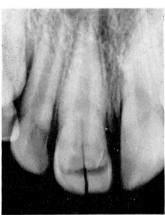

Fig. 427.—Coronal fracture. The cross-shaped fracture of the crown of 1| is due to a vertico-oblique cleavage.

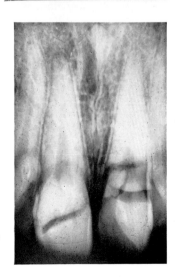

Fig. 428.—Coronal fracture. 1| presents an oblique fracture of the crown. |1 comminuted fracture of the crown involving the cervical portion of the tooth.

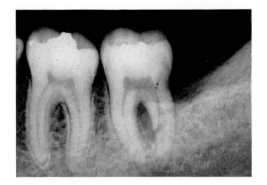

Fig. 429.—Root fracture. Vertical line fracture of the distal root of $\overline{7}$. No displacement of root fragments.

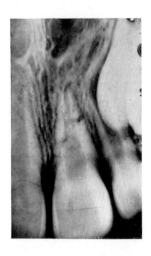

Fig. 430.—Root fracture. Oblique fracture of root of $\underline{|1}$ in socket.

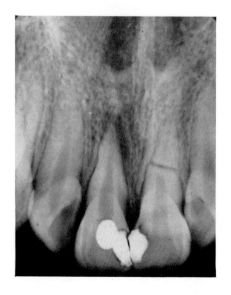

Fig. 431.—Root fracture. Old fracture of middle third of root of $\underline{|1}$. Now united. $\underline{1|}$. Chronic periapical abscess.

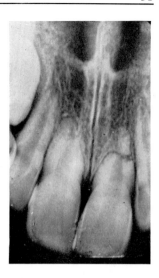

Fig. 432.—Root fracture. Old fracture of the root of |1. Apex separated and fixed in terminal part of the socket.

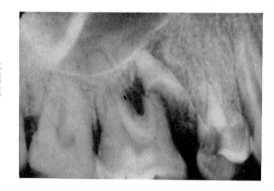

Fig. 433.—Root fracture. Fracture at middle third of mesial root of 6|. Distal fragment displaced into bony interdental septum outside the socket.

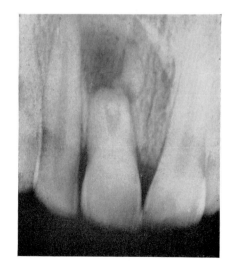

Fig. 434.—Root fracture. 1|. Fractured distal part of root. Apex displaced, and superimposed infection with abscess formation at terminal area of socket.

Fractures of the Jaws and Facial Bones

FRACTURES of the jaws interfere with the opening and closing of the mouth and therefore impair speech and mastication.

These fractures may be considered under the following headings:—

1. The alveolar process.
2. The mandible.
3. The maxilla.
4. The facial bones.

1. The Alveolar Process.—A fracture of the alveolar process is a common occurrence during the extraction of a tooth. It is confined in its site, a small portion only is broken, and the fragments are readily exfoliated.

Following a direct blow on the mouth or a crush accident, much larger areas are involved. The alveolar process becomes one of the many bones fractured.

A pathological fracture of the alveolus is occasionally seen following irradiation of a rodent ulcer of the face, on the lips or cheeks, without the interposition of a protective lead shield.

An alveolar fracture may be seen as a simple linear break or as a comminuted area. After direct violence to the face, extensive portions of the alveolar process are fractured and the fragments may undergo great degrees of displacement, most commonly into the oral cavity. Often, several teeth are carried in a relatively large fragment, which itself can become completely detached from the main bone.

The fracture line may be continuous across the shadow of the teeth and bony interdental septa, and the roots of the teeth are often fractured. A linear fracture is commonly found in the region of the maxillary tuberosity during an attempted extraction of the upper last molar tooth.

When the alveolar fragment separates in the maxillary premolar and molar regions, it carries away part of the floor of the antrum with exposure of the sinus.

2. The Mandible.—The mandible is one of the bones in the body most vulnerable to injury. It is more prone to fracture than the maxilla.

Radiographic examination is indispensable in cases of injury to the mandible, and at least three views should be obtained—postero-anterior, lateral, and occlusal. A comprehensive series of pictures should cover the mandible in its full extent, from condyle to condyle.

A radiographic investigation will determine the presence of a fracture, its site, the amount of displacement and overlapping of the fragments. After reduction, a check can be made by repetitive films of the maintenance of good alinement and the formation of callus.

The medico-legal aspect of every case of fracture must always be borne in mind. The absence of a radiographic examination following an injury to the face promotes an untenable position for the practitioner.

Any part of the mandible may suffer fracture, and it is not uncommon to find two or more breaks in the bone resulting from the same injury. A blow to one side of the chin may produce a fracture at the point of impact and, concurrently, another in the ramus or condylar neck on the opposite side.

A fracture of the mandible may follow direct or indirect violence, or an underlying pathological condition. The break in the bone may be simple, incomplete, compound, or comminuted.

The line of fracture can be vertical or oblique, and the latter either downwards and forwards or downwards and backwards. This line often runs through the socket of erupted or unerupted teeth, and the teeth themselves are sometimes fractured.

The unerupted tooth in its crypt, when lying in the line of fracture, rarely interferes with the progress of union. Retained roots or infected teeth in the path of the separated bone fragments may affect ultimate bone union. The extraction of other teeth in the line of cleavage must be undertaken carefully, lest a simple fracture be converted into a compound one and affect reduction and stabilization of the fragments.

The displacement of the fragments may take place upwards, downwards, inwards, or outwards. The degree and direction depend upon:—

a. Site of the fracture.
b. Direction of the line of fracture.
c. Presence of opposing teeth.
d. Rupture of the periosteum.
e. Muscle pull.
f. Force of the blow.

There is more displacement in the edentulous mandible, particularly when the fractures are bilateral. The bones of the older patient undergo atrophy and become brittle.

Fracture of the Mandible.—The most frequent sites of fracture of the body of the mandible are located between the canine and the angle of the jaw. Fractures at the symphysis are rare. If the line of fracture in this region is vertical there is generally no displacement. The fragments tend to override each other if the line of cleavage is oblique.

The condyle is a common site for a fracture, and the neck or base of the neck is usually involved. The most common causes are indirect violence to the chin, or falling on to one's heels from a great height.

When the fracture of the condyle is unilateral, the head of the condyle is pulled forwards and inwards by the external pterygoid muscle, and may be dislocated if the joint capsule is torn. The lower fragment is pulled upwards and displaced towards the side.

In cases of bilateral condylar fractures, the heads are pulled inwards and forwards, with elevation of the main bone and depression of the chin.

The extracapsular condylar fracture is the more common type, and the high intracapsular variety is often associated with a dislocation of the head in the fossa.

Fractures of the coronoid process are uncommon, and are concurrent with injuries to the maxilla and zygoma. If only the tip is involved, it will probably be retained in its position, but usually the fracture is nearer its base and the fragment is displaced upwards.

Control of the progress of bone union should be undertaken by repetitive radiography with a standard technique. Callus formation often takes several months before it is visible on a radiograph.

After reduction, the fracture area should be observed radiologically with special reference to the following:—

The line of fracture: A slight widening of the gap between the two bone fragments is normal.

Maintenance of alinement of the fragments: No opinion should be submitted unless radiographs are taken in at least two planes. Signs of overriding of the fragments are clearly shown.

Evidence of infection: The edges of the fragments exhibit rarefaction and increased decalcification, with marked irregularity of outline. The line of fracture is widened.

Delayed and non-union: The presence of sequestra is a common cause of delayed union. Non-union is shown to exist when the edges of the fragments become rounded off and cortical bone is deposited at the bone ends.

3. The Maxilla.—

a. The palatal process may be fractured when a hard object or instrument, whilst in the mouth, is driven upwards from below against the palate.

It may be an extension from the alveolar fracture, or be one of the many bones broken in a crush accident or from a major violent facial impact.

Cases have been described where the two halves of the palate were disconnected in the midline in an associated fracture.

b. The body of the maxilla, enclosing the antrum, suffers a fracture from a direct blow upon the zygomatic area of the face. The antral wall becomes comminuted and the zygoma is usually depressed into the antral cavity.

Accidents of the maxilla are generally associated with fractures of the malar and nasal bones. The maxillary sinuses are commonly filled with blood, and infection of the sinuses is not an unusual complication.

A common fracture of the maxilla has been described which extends horizontally across the body of the bone between the floor of the maxillary sinuses and the floor of the orbits. The lower segment of the maxilla may be completely detached from its base.

Maxillary fractures invariably heal by fibrous and not by osseous union.

4. The Facial Bones.—

a. Nasal Bones.—These bones are extremely prone to fracture. The injury varies from a simple linear fracture to a comminuted fracture with severe depression of the nasal crest. Often there is lateral displacement of the nasal bones with fracture of the nasal process of the maxilla.

b. Zygomatic Arch.—Direct violence usually results in comminution and depression of the bone. The weakest part of the arch is the synchondrosis between the zygomatic process of the temporal bone and the temporal process of the malar bone.

c. Malar Bone.—Fracture of the body of the malar bone is rare. The star-shaped malar body tends to rotate upon its maxillary process when subject to a severe blow.

The three remaining processes, the frontal, the infra-orbital, and the temporal, may fracture or loosen at their respective synchondroses and produce wide gaps at these points.

A fracture along the infra-orbital margin is generally situated in the region of the infra-orbital foramen and not at the synchondrosis. The floor of the orbit is tilted and raised in this area and may damage the eyeball.

A unilateral fracture of the malar bone due to indirect violence may compound into the maxillary sinus.

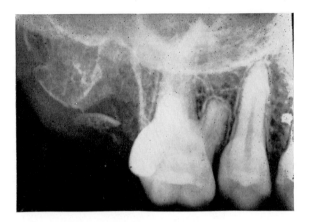

Fig. 435.—Fracture of the alveolar process. Empty $\underline{8|}$ socket after extraction of the last upper right molar tooth. Much alveolar fragmentation has resulted.

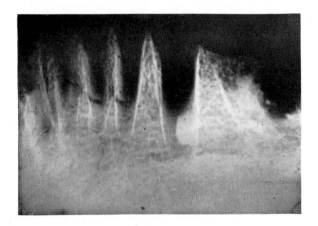

Fig. 436.—$\overline{21|12}$. Alveolar fracture during extraction of the teeth.

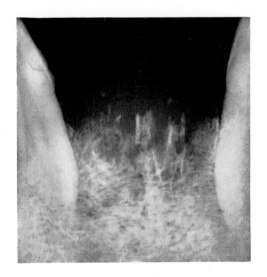

Fig. 437.—$\overline{21|12}$. Gross comminuted alveolar fracture with destructive osteitis.

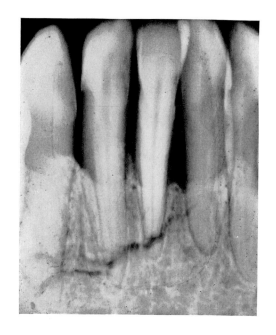

Fig. 438.—Oblique fracture of the alveolar process in $\overline{321|1}$ region as a result of a direct blow. The apices of $\overline{21|}$ are fractured. Old-standing marginal periodontitis with recession of the bone.

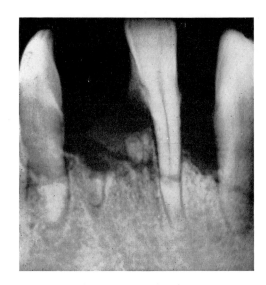

Fig. 439.—Comminuted fracture of the alveolar process in $\overline{21|12}$ region. Apex retained in $\overline{1|}$ socket. Alveolar fragmentation in $\overline{21|}$ area. Fracture of the distal part of root $\overline{|2}$.

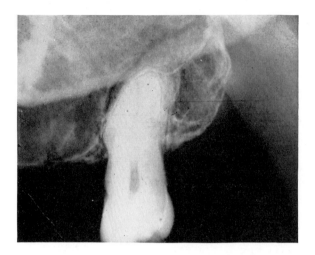

Fig. 440.—Cleavage of the maxillary tuberosity while attempting extraction of the upper left third molar tooth.

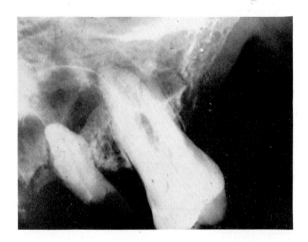

Fig. 441.—Fracture of the alveolar process in the |5̱6̱ region after a direct blow. The alveolar fragment carrying root |5̱ and the |6̱ has separated from the maxilla, exposing the floor of the antrum.

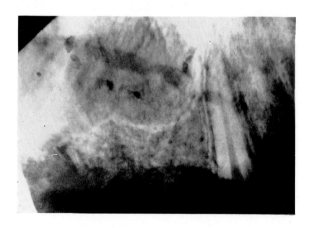

Fig. 442.—Fracture of the alveolar process in the 7̱6̱5̱4̱3̱| region. The line of fracture runs through the lower third of the right antrum.

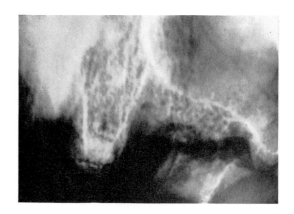

Fig. 443.—Fractured alveolus in edentulous |45 region. The alveolar fragment is completely detached from the main bone and is displaced downwards.

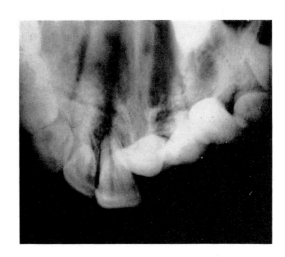

Fig. 444.—Alveolar fracture in 4321|1234 area. The alveolar process in the |1234 is not detached from the maxilla but is displaced into the oral cavity.

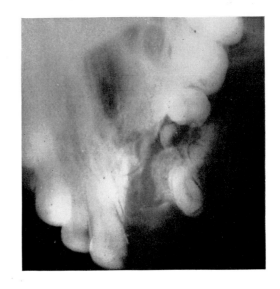

Fig. 445.—Direct violence has fractured the alveolar process in the |1234 region. The fragment carrying roots and a tooth is totally separated from the maxilla.

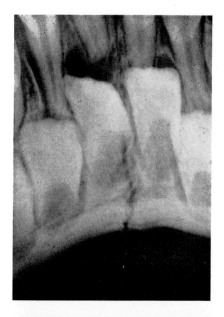

Fig. 446.—Symphysis menti. Fracture in the lower central region in child, aged 4 years, who fell on chin. The midline synchondrosis has given way. The symphysis unites at the end of the first year of life.

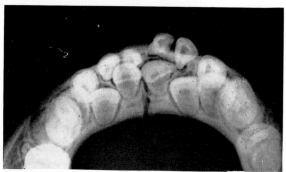

Fig. 447.—Occlusal view of *Fig.* 446. Limited separation and gap between the two halves of the mandible. No deformity, and good alinement.

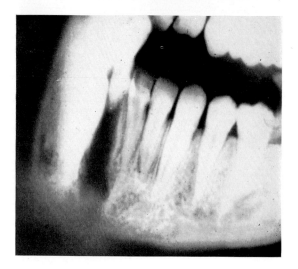

Fig. 448.—Lateral oblique view of a fracture in the midline of the mandible. Excellent visualization with limited distortion.

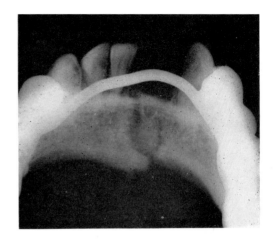

Fig. 449.—Comminuted fracture at the symphysis menti. Reduced to good alinement and maintained in position by splinting.

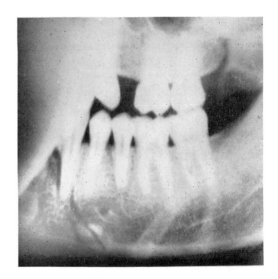

Fig. 450.—Canine region. Oblique fracture line running downwards and outwards from the alveolar margin between the left lateral incisor and canine teeth. The fracture is of the complete variety as it has penetrated the lower border of the mandible. No displacements of fragments. The socket of the canine is involved, but there is no fracture of the root of the tooth.

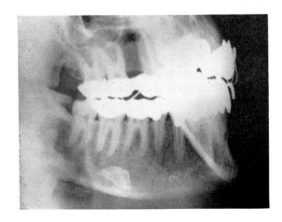

Fig. 451.—Premolar region. The line of fracture is directed almost vertically downwards between the right lower premolar teeth. The break in the bone has not reached the lower border of the mandible, and is termed an incomplete fracture. The bifurcation of the fracture line is a radiographic illusion, due to the superimposition of the two edges of the oblique fracture—the broken inner and outer walls of the mandible.

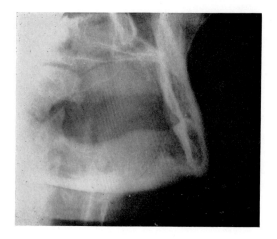

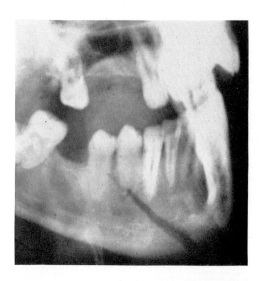

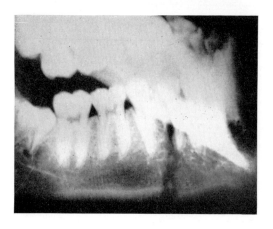

Fig. 452.—An incomplete fracture in the right mandibular premolar region. The line of fracture is directed downwards and backwards.

Fig. 453.—The fracture extends downwards and forwards from the right premolar region through the lower border of the mandible. The posterior part of the body of the mandible is displaced downwards, leaving a wide gap at the site of the fracture.

Fig. 454.—The fracture in the premolar region is vertical in direction. The gap between the two edges of the bone contains sequestra, which often are a cause of delayed bone union.

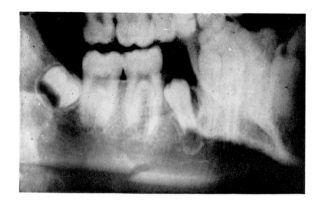

Fig. 455.—The downward and backward line of fracture runs through the crypt of the unerupted lower right second premolar tooth. The apical part of the crypt socket has been severed.

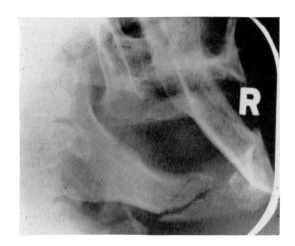

Fig. 456.—A comminuted fracture in the premolar region of the mandible in an edentulous patient. Fractures of the body of the mandible are more likely to be compound into the mouth or to the outside of the face.

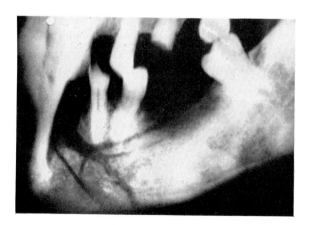

Fig. 457.—Gross comminuted fracture in the left premolar region. The separated large alveolar fragment is carrying the two premolar teeth in their sockets.

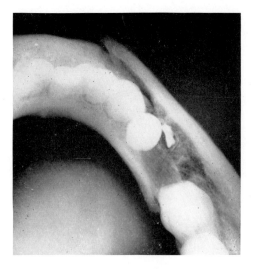

Fig. 458.—An occlusal view of a fracture in the premolar region. The obliquity of the line of fracture is seen running across the transverse axis of the mandible from outer to inner walls.

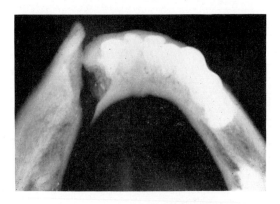

Fig. 459.—The overriding of the fragments is demonstrated. There is lingual displacement of the main part of the mandible.

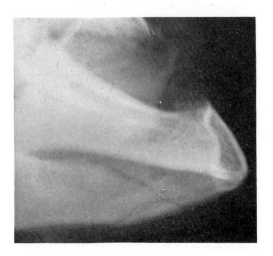

Fig. 460.—The radiating lines of fracture in the premolar region of the mandible have not produced any separation or displacement of the bone fragments. This is probably due to the periosteum remaining intact.

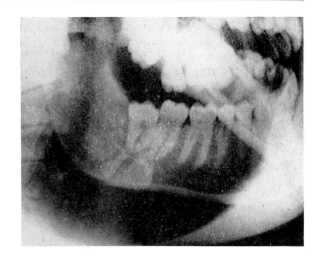

Fig. 461.—An incomplete fracture extending from the apices of the unerupted |8̄ downwards and backwards just short of the lower border of the mandible. This occurred during the attempted extraction of the tooth.

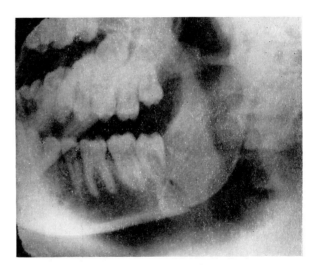

Fig. 462.—A complete fracture similar to that in *Fig.* 461.

Fig. 463.—This fracture in the left molar-angle region followed the attempt at surgical removal of the |8̄ roots. Local chronic osteitis and abscess formation around the roots of |7̄8̄ had produced a rarefying condition of the immediate bone structure.

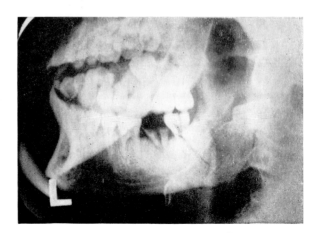

14

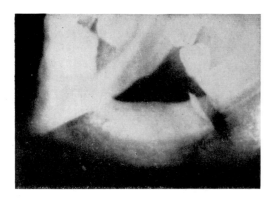

Fig. 464.—At operation for the removal of the $\overline{8}$, the tooth was split and a complete fracture resulted.

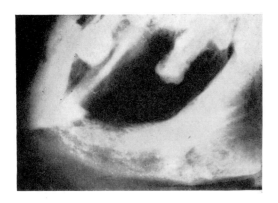

Fig. 465.—Strong, dense bone union of the fracture shown in *Fig.* 464, in good alinement, five months later.

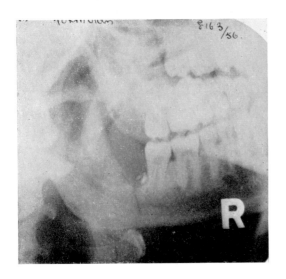

Fig. 466.—Incomplete fracture during surgical removal of unerupted horizontally impacted $\overline{8|}$.

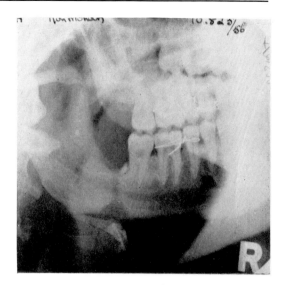

Fig. 467.—Same as *Fig.* 466. Within four weeks, a superimposed infection brought about a complete pathological fracture, with much rarefying osteitis spreading to the lower border of the mandible and widening of gap between the fragments.

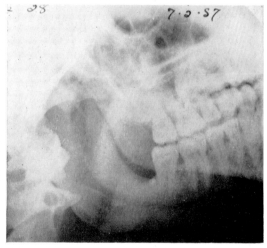

Fig. 468.—Same as *Figs.* 466, 467. Complete bone union, with no signs of sclerosis, after antibiotic treatment, six months after the production of the fracture. The retention of the apposing molar teeth has assisted in maintaining good alinement.

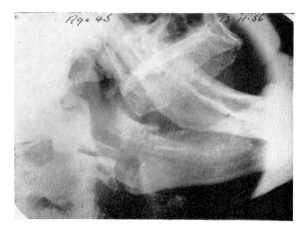

Fig. 469.—Angle of mandible. Oblique fracture at the angle of the jaw following a motor-car accident. The ramus is slightly elevated and there is some overriding of the fragments.

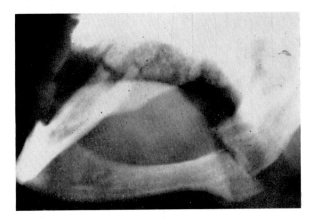

Fig. 470.—Oblique fracture at the angle of the mandible in an edentulous patient, as a result of a blow on the chin. There is much displacement and marked elevation of the ramus.

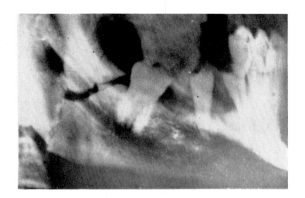

Fig. 471.—Right-angled fracture in the molar-angle region. The direction of the fracture lines is of importance in this region, as it plays a vital part in maintaining the posterior fragment in the correct position.

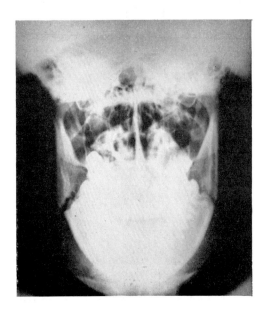

Fig. 472.—Bilateral angular fracture with no apparent displacement of the mandible or rami.

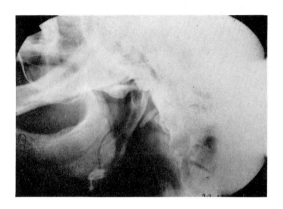

Fig. 473.—Ramus. Bifurcated fracture extending downwards from the mandibular notch, branching to below the base of the condyle and to the angle of the jaw.

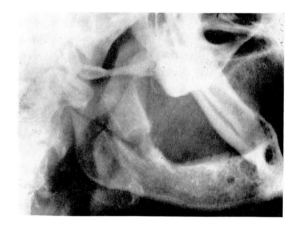

Fig. 474.—Comminuted fracture of the ascending ramus. The main fracture line extends downwards and forwards from the base of the condylar process to the lower part of the anterior border of the ramus. The coronoid process is separated by the oblique fracture.

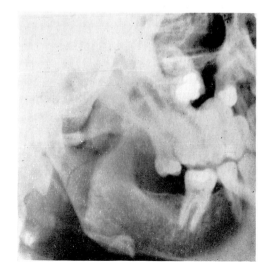

Fig. 475.—Oblique fracture at the base of the condylar process. No displacement of the fragments.

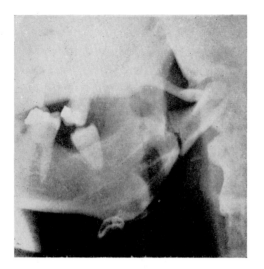

Fig. 476.—Similar fracture to that shown in *Fig.* 475. Sequestra lying between the fragments. The main part of the mandible is retained in good position by the apposing last molar teeth. The condylar process is displaced slightly forwards.

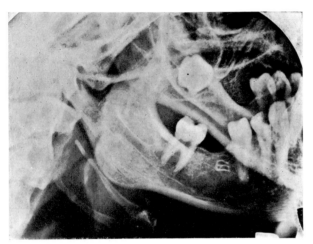

Fig. 477.—Oblique fracture at the base of the condyle. The mandible is elevated, and the condyle is overriding it.

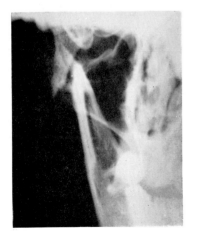

Fig. 478.—Postero-anterior view of *Fig.* 477. This shows that in addition to the overriding of the condylar process, the latter is displaced outwards.

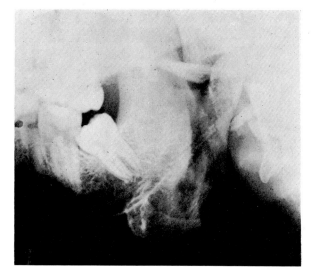

Fig. 479.—Crack just below the condylar head. No displacement of the head or ramus.

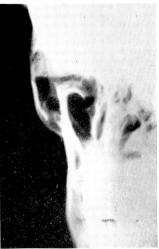

Fig. 480.—Fracture at the neck of the condylar process. Forward dislocation of the condylar head.

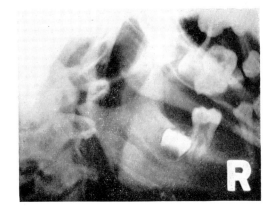

Fig. 481.—Intracapsular fracture of the condylar head. Forward dislocation of the head. This type of fracture is not common.

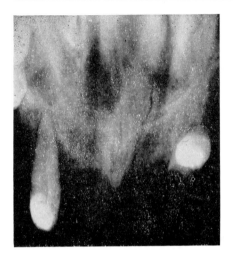

Fig. 482.—Fracture of the palatal process. Linear crack in the left palatal process, extending backwards almost parallel with the midline suture.

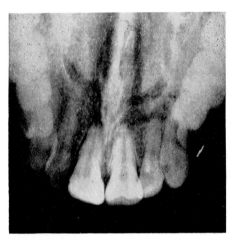

Fig. 483.—Comminuted fracture of the anterior part of both palatal processes, with communication to and through the nasal fossæ.

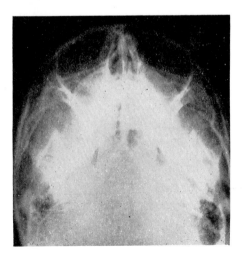

Fig. 484.—Depressed fracture of the left zygomatic arch following a direct blow.

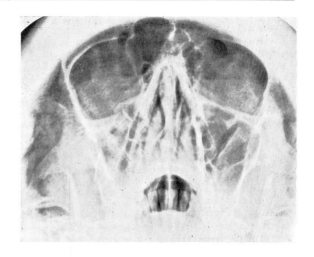

Fig. 485.—Postero-anterior view of fracture of the infra-orbital margin of the right orbit. Depression and comminution of the external margin.

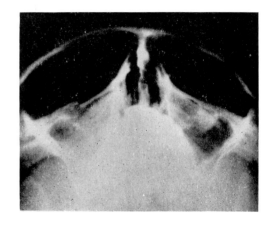

Fig. 486.—Tangential view of a fracture of the infra-orbital margin of the right orbit. The outer part of the floor is pushed upwards into the orbit.

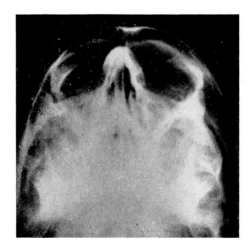

Fig. 487.—Postero-anterior view of a comminuted fracture of the right malar bone. The maxillary process of the frontal bone is fractured and the frontomalar synchondrosis is open.

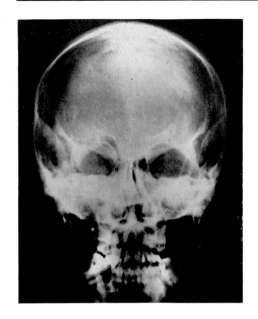

Fig. 488.—Postero-anterior view of Fig. 487.

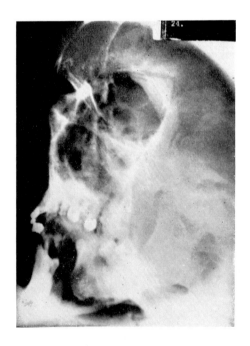

Fig. 489.—Oblique lateral view of Fig. 487. The frontomalar processes are clearly shown fractured.

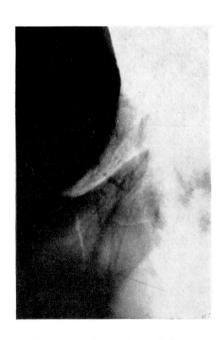

Fig. 490.—Comminuted fracture of the nasal bones.

Pathological Fractures

PATHOLOGICAL fractures of the teeth and jaws are not common.

A pathological fracture is a break in the tooth or bone, the structure of which has been changed and attenuated by atrophy of disuse, advanced age, or by disease.

Although any factor which weakens or destroys the bone may be regarded as a predisposing condition, the actual determining factor is a blow or muscular action. The force of the blow may be slight, and may occur in cases of an accident otherwise insufficient to break the jaw.

Idiopathic resorption of the root of a tooth, whether originating in the pulp of the tooth or at the periphery, may involve the complete internal structure. The wall of the crown becomes extremely thin and weakened, and a fracture may follow while masticating hard food. The break is usually subgingival in position.

A local rarefying osteitis arising from an infected tooth or root may spread centrifugally into the main bone, destroying the bone in its wake. In the mandible, the destruction may spread from wall to wall or from the alveolar margin to its lower border.

A large abscess cavity or trough may form, containing sequestra. If drainage of the pus is not effected, the condition will progress and a pathological fracture will result to set up its own method of evacuation of the pus.

Osteomyelitis is much more common in the mandible than in the maxilla. The entire bone may be involved and result in sequestration of a major part of the bone. With the use in modern times of chemotherapy, the destructive process is more readily arrested, but occasionally a pathological fracture results from minor and unexpected trauma. Tertiary syphilitic osteomyelitis may also produce changes in the bone which may readily suffer cleavage following slight trauma.

Spontaneous fracture in cases of cysts, even of large size, is extremely rare. On the other hand, the presence of a large cyst in the bone predisposes it to pathological fracture from minor injury. Fractures caused by odontogenic cysts are not so rare.

Benign tumours in and around the mouth do not produce spontaneous fractures, nor do primary malignant growths. The mandible is a common site of metastatic deposits from primary carcinoma in other parts of the body and is prone to pathological fracture. Occasionally, the maxilla and palate exhibit a fracture due to the extension of a sarcoma from the antrum.

Irradiation of malignant tumours of the jaw is contra-indicated and usually leads to radio-necrosis and a pathological fracture.

Pathological fractures are also found in skeletal conditions involving the mandible and maxilla, such as osteogenesis imperfecta, myelomatosis, and Paget's disease.

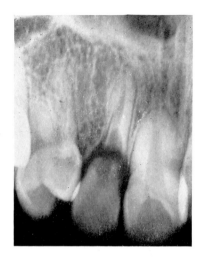

Fig. 491.—The proximal half of the pulp canal in 2| shows an elongated dilatation produced by internal resorption of the root. The dentine and cementum have been eroded from within, culminating in a transverse pathological fracture of the root in this region.

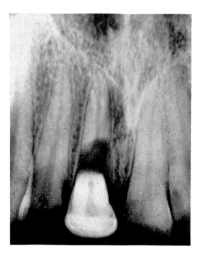

Fig. 492.—Pathological fracture of 1| due to internal resorption of the root in its middle third. Osseous metaplastic changes are seen in the punched-out radiolucent area.

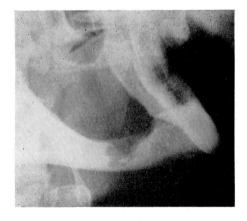

Fig. 493.—Root fragment and sequestra in area of destructive osteitis in large abscess cavity in 6| region. The bone destruction is proceeding towards the lower border of the mandible with a pathological fracture imminent.

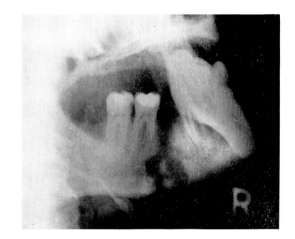

Fig. 494.—The lower right second premolar tooth has been extracted, but bone necrosis has extended to and through the inferior border of the mandible, causing a pathological fracture with sequestra in the area of fracture.

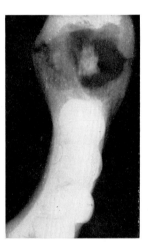

Fig. 495.—Irregular sequestrum lying in abscess area in $\overline{|345}$ region. Owing to lack of effective drainage of the pus, a pathological fracture has ensued across the mandible from inner to outer wall.

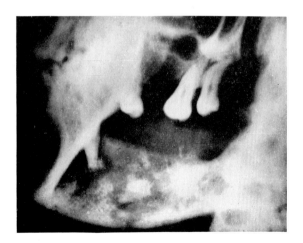

Fig. 496.—Osteomyelitis in $\overline{|1-7}$ region with sequestrum formation and pathological fracture.

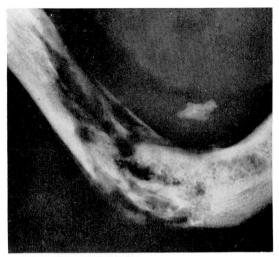

Fig. 497.—Occlusal view of the
right mandible showing widespread osteomyelitis. Sequestra
have been thrown off into the
soft tissue of the floor of the
mouth. A pathological fracture
may occur at any moment.

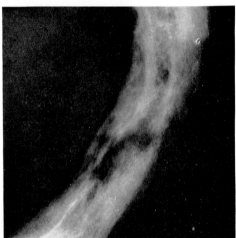

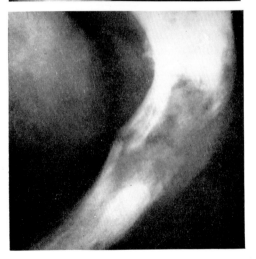

Figs. 498, 499.—Long-standing osteomyelitis of the left mandible. The
destructive process is involving the
$\overline{1-7}$ area with eventual pathological
fracture.

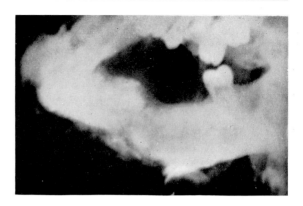

Fig. 500.—Active osteomyelitis involving the whole of the left mandible with a pathological fracture.

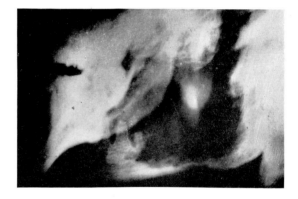

Fig. 501.—$\overline{|5-8}$. The active osteomyelitis has subsided with the shedding of a large part of the mandible as sequestra. The lower border of the mandible is almost on the point of a pathological fracture.

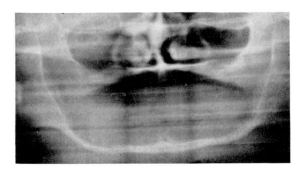

Fig. 502.—A rotograph of the mandible showing abnormal degree of bone resorption. The atrophy of the bone predisposes it to a pathological fracture.

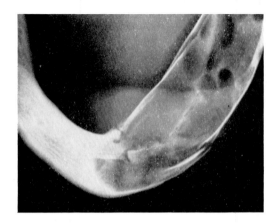

Fig. 503.—Occlusal view showing a multilocular dental cyst extending from the midline along the body of the left mandible to the molar region. There is a pathological fracture running across the anterior part of the cystic lesion.

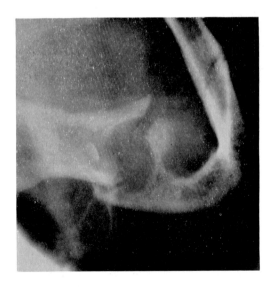

Fig. 504.—External lateral oblique view of the body of the left mandible, showing a pathological fracture through a large cyst in the left premolar region.

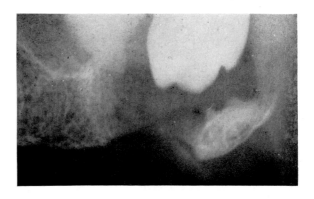

Fig. 505.—Unerupted |8 in a dentigerous cyst which has distended, carrying the bone of the tuberosity away in its wall. A pathological fracture has occurred.

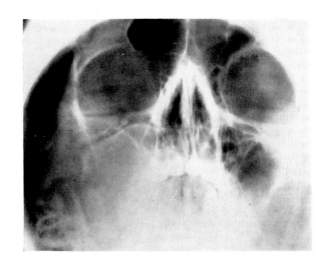

Fig. 506.—A cystic odontome occupying the entire right maxillary sinus and producing a pathological fracture of the right infra-orbital plate.

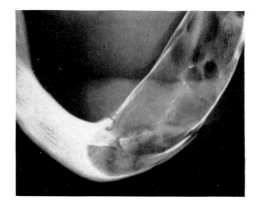

Fig. 507.—Pathological fracture across a large multilocular periodontal cyst in the mandible.

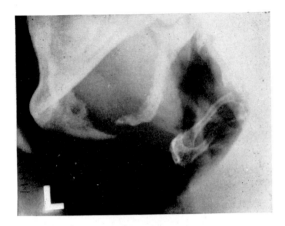

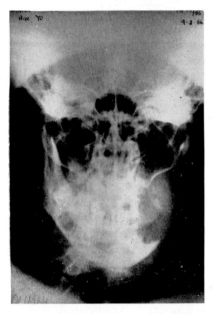

Figs. 508, 509.—Gross invasion of the bony mandible extending from the left canine region to the left coronoid process, with a pathological fracture. The original condition was a malignant neoplasm of the gingiva.

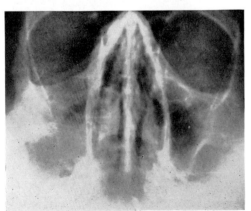

Fig. 510.—Malignant growth, arising in the right maxillary antrum, which has destroyed the whole of the outer wall of the antrum.

The Maxillary Antrum

THE alveolar process of the upper jaw, carrying the roots of the maxillary teeth, forms the floor of the antrum of Highmore. This anatomical relationship establishes a common ground and close interest for the dental surgeon, the facio-maxillary surgeon, and the rhinologist.

Lesions involving the maxillary teeth frequently encroach upon and penetrate into the antrum. Conversely, pathological conditions arising in the antrum or from its walls may extend down to the tooth-bearing area of the upper jaw.

Radiographic examination is of the utmost importance in this particular field. Changes in the translucency of the cavity and in the contour and continuity of the antral walls are easily discerned.

An increase in the antral density may be produced by inflammatory œdema of the mucosal lining, by accumulation of mucus, blood, or pus in the antral cavity, and by internal or invading new growth formations. Distension of the bony walls may be caused by invading and expanding odontogenic cysts and by the proliferation of benign tumours.

Erosion and destruction of the antral walls may result from osteomyelitis and from extension of malignant neoplasms.

Opacities of the maxillary antrum may be considered as follows:—

1. Superimposed shadows.
2. Marginal shadows.
3. Basal shadows.
4. Total opacity.
5. Foreign bodies.

Changes in the antral walls are seen as:—

1. Expansion and distension.
2. Erosion and destruction.

1. Superimposed Shadows are cast upon the radiographic image of the antra by opaque or semi-opaque swellings, embedded or embodied in the soft tissue or bone structure in or around the antra. These opacities will appear on the film if they are in the direct line of the X-ray beam which is being concentrated upon the antra.

The most common superimposed shadows are those of:—

a. Petrous bone.
b. Upper lip.
c. Malar bone.
d. Facial œdema.
e. Foreign bodies.

2. Marginal Shadows are depicted as irregular, peripheral, hazy opacities continuous with the inner surface of the antral walls. They do not obliterate the antral cavity.

Such shadows may be produced by:—

a. Sinusitis.
b. Polypoid formations.
c. Rhinoliths.
d. Benign new growths.
e. Cysts.

3. Basal Shadows are identified as opacities concentrated on the floor of the antrum and in the lower part of the sinus. The contour of the upper limit of these shadows may be an important diagnostic feature. A horizontal fluid level usually indicates an antral effusion or empyema, while an upward convexity is the delineation of a cyst or granuloma. These opacities may represent:—

a. Empyemas.
b. Extravasation of blood.
c. Polypoid formations.
d. Osteomas.
e. Granulomas and cysts.

4. Total Opacity of the Antrum is due to obliteration of the sinus cavity. It is often impossible to determine the underlying pathological condition, but the following conditions may be responsible:—

a. Empyema.
b. Neoplasms.
c. Hyperostosis.
d. Cystic odontomes.

5. Foreign Bodies may be located in the antrum. They may lie on the floor beneath the mucosa without gaining access to the sinus cavity. Others penetrate into the antrum. Infection of the maxillary sinus is a common complication. The foreign bodies may include:—

a. Root fragments.
b. Pieces of shrapnel.
c. Air-gun pellets.

Changes in the Antral Walls.—Certain lesions cause the antrum to expand its walls, others destroy the bony walls.

Expansion and distension result from the growth of benign neoplasms within the sinus cavity or from enlargement of cystic formations.

Erosion and destruction of the antral walls are concomitant with infiltrating malignant conditions and with extensive osteomyelitis.

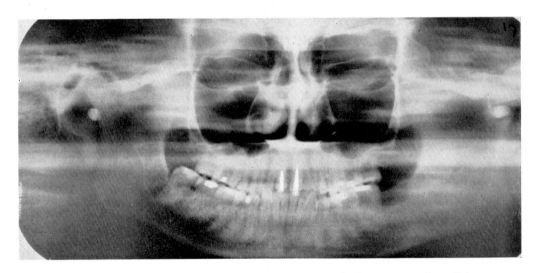

Fig. 511.—The rotographic view presents a truer anatomical representation of the antrum than by the routine postero-anterior technique. Both the antero-external and postero-external surfaces are shown in the same plane.

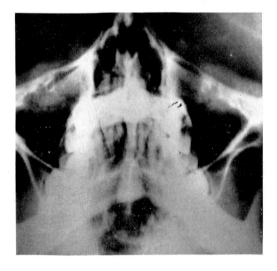

Fig. 512.—The routine postero-anterior radiographic view depicts the maxillary sinus as a dark, radiolucent, inverted triangular area below the orbit and above the upper premolar and molar teeth. It is bounded by the external wall of the nasal fossa on the inner aspect and by a well-defined, sharp, peripheral, heavy, thick, white line on its outer limit. The two sinuses are usually symmetrical in size and shape.

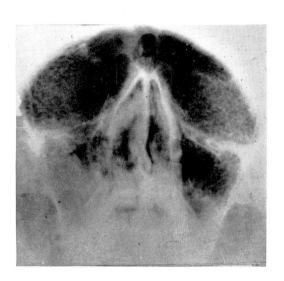

Fig. 513.—The right antrum reveals a peripheral hazy opacity, of varying thickness, due to hyperæmic swelling of the lining mucosa. When the inflammatory condition subsides, the marginal shadowing disappears. If the infection persists, mucus and pus may form and accumulate in the cavity as an empyema.

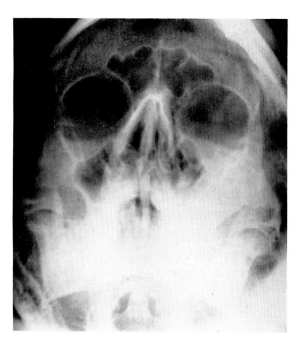

Fig. 514.—The left antrum shows a thickening of its outer wall. The diffuse, marginal, dense opacity is produced by a local hyperostosis of the postero-external surface of the maxilla.

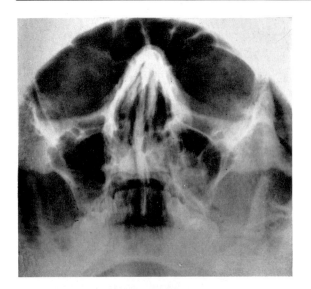

Fig. 515.—There is an indefinite cloudiness, ovoid in shape, in the vertical axis, masking the inner part of the image of the antrum. It is a superimposed external shadow of cellulitis of the soft tissue of the face and buccal sulcus, associated with a periapical lesion of the upper left canine and premolar teeth.

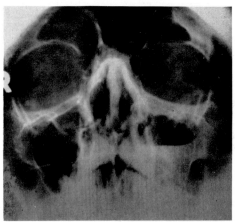

Fig. 516.—Empyema in the left antrum. Uniform, cone-shaped opacity, occupying the lower part of the left antrum, with a well-defined upper horizontal fluid level. The formation of pus in the sinus usually follows upon an acute or chronic sinusitis, from a periapical infection of an underlying maxillary tooth, or from the perforation of a suppurating cyst which has entered the antrum.

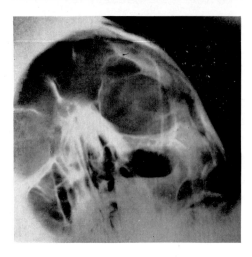

Fig. 517.—The head is tilted to the right, and the fluid level of the pus in the left antrum assumes a new horizontal position. This is an important diagnostic feature.

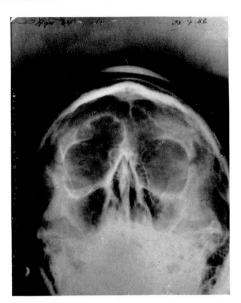

Fig. 518.—The left malar bone is fractured, showing widening of the fronto-malar synchondrosis and separation at the malar-zygomatic junction. The cloudiness in the outer part of the left antrum is due to hæmorrhage into the sinus caused by tearing of the mucosa.

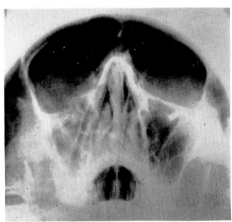

Fig. 519.—There is a fracture of the right maxillary complex involving the floor of the right orbit. The hazy opacity of the right antrum represents the collection of blood in the sinus. There is no fluid level. If the blood-clot becomes infected, the shadow will increase in density and develop a well-defined upper horizontal limit.

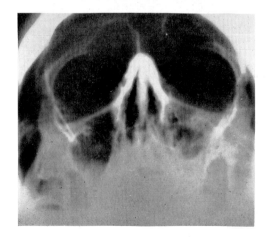

Fig. 520.—At the base of the right maxillary sinus there is a globular mass of low opacity. It is a polypoid formation due to a localized thickening of the basal mucosa after a prolonged attack of sinusitis.

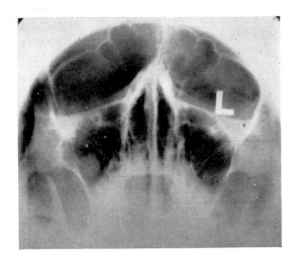

Fig. 521.—Lateral type of polypoid formation arising from the outer wall of the right antrum, on its inner aspect. It appears to be pedunculated.

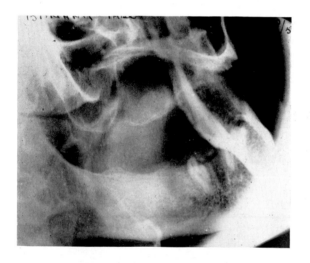

Fig. 522.—A dome-shaped, sessile opacity is arising from the floor of the antrum. It is an osteoma, benign in character, and exhibits cancellous bone structure.

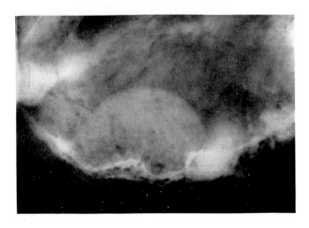

Fig. 523.—Posterior to the basal osteoma is the retained root of |8. The cloudiness of the antral shadow is indicative of an associated secondary infection of the maxillary sinus.

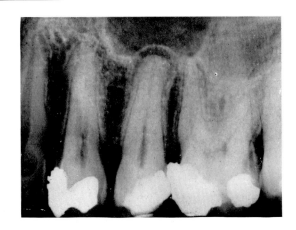

Fig. 524.—There is a small epithe-liated granuloma in connexion with the |5. It is seen slightly invaginating the floor of the antrum.

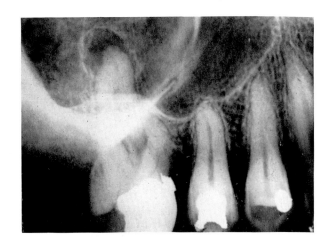

Fig. 525.—Larger granu-loma around the 6| pene-trating the antrum.

Fig. 526.—The lesion in con-nexion with the retained roots |67 is a developing periodontal cyst. It has entered the left maxillary sinus and is located at its floor, and its translucency is in keeping with non-suppurative contents.

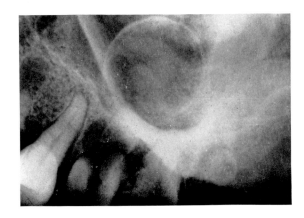

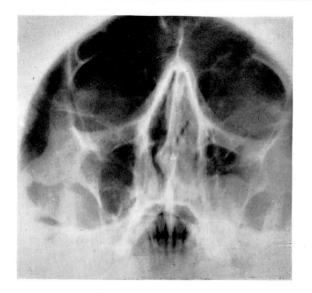

Fig. 527.—Postero-anterior view of same patient as in Fig. 526 five months later. The roots were extracted after the first radiographic examination but the patient refused the removal of the cyst. The cyst has grown larger, and the increased opacity indicates that the content is pus.

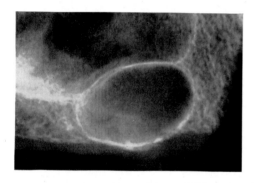

Fig. 528.—Residual periodontal cyst in edentulous molar region elevating the floor of the antrum into its own cavity.

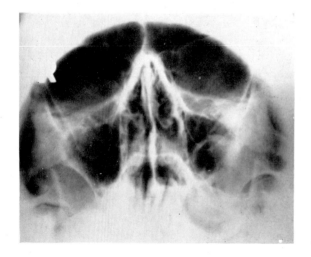

Fig. 529.—Periodontal cyst which has penetrated into the left maxillary sinus.

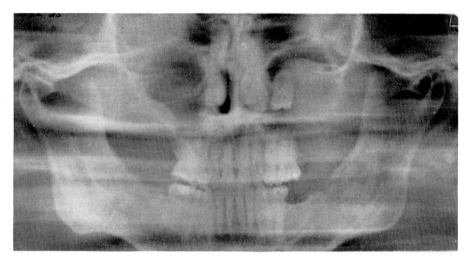

Fig. 530.—Rotograph showing large dentigerous cyst with an unerupted tooth occupying almost the whole cavity of the left sinus.

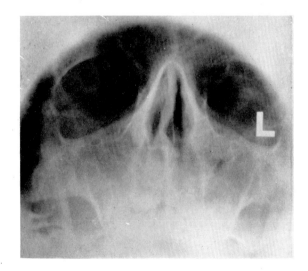

Fig. 531.—Both antra are completely filled with fluid or pus and present a white, uniform opacity. There is no indication of the identity of the underlying cause.

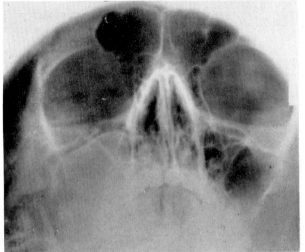

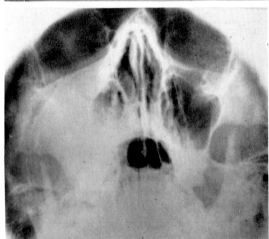

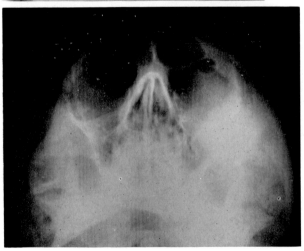

Fig. 532.—The whole of the right sinus cavity is occupied by a large cystic odontome. At the lower part of the antrum, on its outer border, there is a collection of denticles, with a loss of the bony wall at this site.

Fig. 533.—Complete obliteration of the right sinus cavity by an osteoma involving the body of the right maxilla and malar bone.

Fig. 534.—Complete obliteration of the left sinus cavity by an osteoma involving the body of the left maxilla, the malar bone, the outer wall of the left orbit, and the great wing of the sphenoid bone.

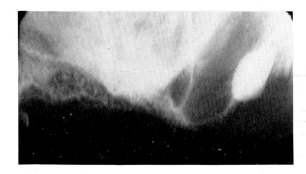

Fig. 535.—Intra-oral view of a root fragment in the 6| region lying at the floor of the left antrum. The fragment is lying in the mucosa and has not found access into the sinus cavity.

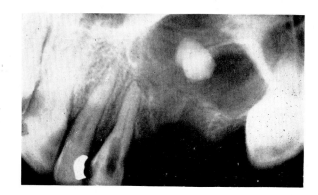

Fig. 536.—Root fragment lying loosely in the left maxillary sinus.

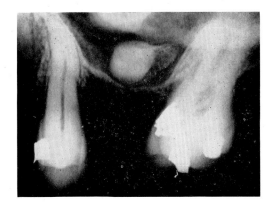

Fig. 537.—The root fragment of the |6 has penetrated into the left antrum. It is lying loosely in the sinus cavity and may change its position with movement of the head.

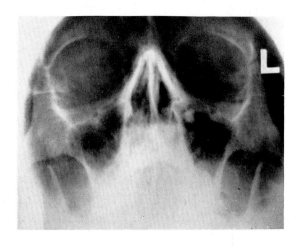

Figs. 538, 539.—Postero-anterior and lateral oblique views of a root fragment pushed into the left antrum during the extraction of the |5. The fragment has travelled to the roof of the sinus cavity and is lying just below the orbital floor at the nasal wall.

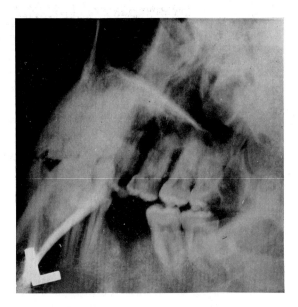

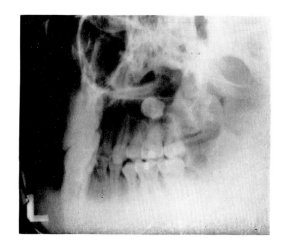

Fig. 540.—Root fragment of the ⌊8 has penetrated into the left maxillary antrum and is lying on the floor of the sinus. The apical part of the upper last molar socket is open and communicates with the antrum, creating an oro-antral fistula.

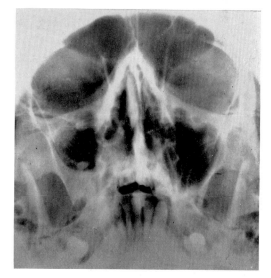

Fig. 541.—Retained root fragment in right antrum lying on an empyema. Infection of the maxillary sinus containing a root fragment is not an uncommon occurrence.

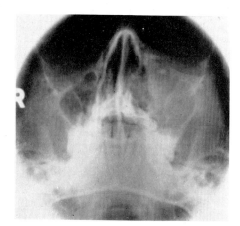

Fig. 542.—The outer wall of the left maxillary sinus is distended by a cystic odontome which is filling the cavity completely. The unerupted denticle is just below the left orbit, whose floor is uplifted into the orbital cavity.

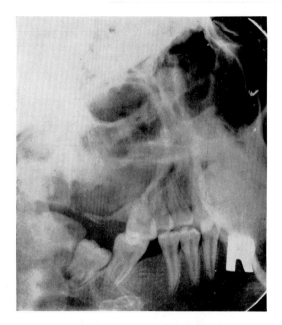

Fig. 543.—Lateral oblique view of the right maxillary sinus which is completely occupied by an expanding cystic odontome. The walls of the right sinus are distended.

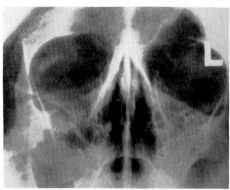

Fig. 544.—Bilateral chronic sinusitis, with total opacity of the antra, and chronic osteomyelitis. The floor of the right orbit and the walls of the right antrum have been destroyed by direct involvement from the internal sinusitis. Active sequestration can be seen.

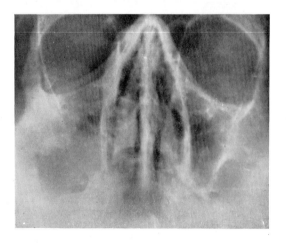

Fig. 545.—Carcinoma of the mucosa of the right maxillary sinus. The inner and outer walls of the right sinus, in their lower halves, have been destroyed by the infiltrating tumour tissue.

PART III

CYSTS AND NEW GROWTHS INVOLVING TEETH, JAWS,
AND SOFT TISSUES

I.—Cysts of the Jaw

1. Follicular or odontogenic cysts.
2. Periodontal or radicular cysts.
3. Traumatic cysts.
4. Non-odontogenic cysts.

Cysts of the Jaw

Cysts of the jaw are of most frequent occurrence. The diagnosis as to the particular variety of cyst, however, should not be made on the radiograph alone.

A circumscribed radiolucent area seen in the maxilla or mandible is, at most, indicative of loss of local bone tissue. The actual shadow cannot reveal whether the condition has been caused by local resorption of bone, whether it has arisen from the proliferation of the dental lamina, from the enamel organ of a developing tooth, or from enclaved epithelial cell rests.

The final diagnosis must be left to the histopathologist. His conclusions depend upon the presence of a fibrous capsule, the existence of an epithelial lining, the association with dental structures, and the examination of the contents of the cyst.

In the determination of the lesion, radiography is of the greatest possible value. The radiograph will show the size and site of the cyst, its relation to the standing teeth, and its connexion or encroachment upon the normal anatomical structures in the jaws.

Much may be deduced from the general outline of the radiolucent area, its definition, its regularity, and its cortical envelopment. The internal image of the cystic area is often of significance, with its varying density, trabeculated character, and septal formation. The amount of cystic fluid and the pressure it exerts cause distension and expansion of the bone, and the degree of bone expansion may be an important clue in differential diagnosis, not only between different types of cysts, but of similar and allied lesions.

The radiograph will show the extension of a cyst into the maxillary sinus, into the nasal cavity, through the floor of the mouth, and may show pressure upon, or displacement of, the inferior dental canal or posterior palatine foramen. Injection of a radio-opaque substance into the cyst lumen is often employed in the delineation of the outline of the cyst.

There are a number of soft-tissue tumours whose radiographic shadows may simulate the image of a cyst of the jaw. Even wide experience and careful examination cannot differentiate cystic formations from lesions such as ameloblastomata, central fibromata, myxomata, benign giant-cell tumours, and osteoclastomata.

Any form of cyst may be multiple, multilocular, or bilateral.

Follicular or Odontogenic Cysts

FOLLICULAR cysts arise from the odontogenic epithelium or tooth follicle and contain part of an unerupted tooth within their sacs.

The following types are recognized:—

1. Eruption Cysts occur on teeth about to erupt and are found in the young patient immediately below the gum surface. They are seen most often associated with unerupted canines and third molar teeth. The upper border of the cyst, pushing its way through the oral margin, rarely casts a shadow on the radiograph.

2. Central Dentigerous Cysts are large eruption cysts formed around the crowns of the teeth. Often the whole of a fully-formed tooth may be found within the cyst. There is no change in the normal enamel formation.

3. Lateral Dentigerous Cysts form at the side of the crown of an unerupted tooth and are commonly found on the distal side of partly erupted third molar teeth. These particular types of cysts tend to extend upwards into the ascending ramus, sometimes reaching as far as the mandibular notch. In the incisor and premolar regions, the unerupted teeth associated with a lateral dentigerous cyst may be displaced vertically downwards to the periphery of the jaw, or obliquely across the alveolar process away from the line of occlusion.

4. Primordial or Simple Follicular Cysts are formed before the formation of the tooth enamel and therefore do not contain any dental structure. They are not common lesions, and are found during routine radiographic examination in young adults in the third molar region and ascending ramus. They are often multilocular, and may develop from the tooth follicle of a supernumerary third molar tooth.

Dentigerous cysts occur in both jaws and may be associated with any tooth or combination of teeth, in both dentitions or with supernumerary teeth. Although they are lesions of adolescence, dentigerous cysts may not be detected until late in adult life and in patients otherwise completely edentulous.

Radiographically they present circular radiolucent areas with well-defined rounded cortical circumferences, containing part or most of an unerupted tooth. They produce much bone expansion and tend to extend along the long axis of the jaws. Multiloculation is a common feature, causing difficulty in differentiating them from adamantinomas.

In their growth they are responsible for tooth displacement, and the radiograph will determine their location. Dentigerous cysts carrying unerupted teeth occasionally invade the antrum.

Secondary infection of dentigerous cysts is not uncommon.

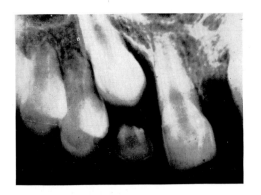

Fig. 546.—Eruption cyst in connexion with unerupted 3|.

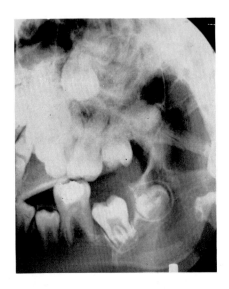

Fig. 547.—Eruption cyst around unerupted |7.

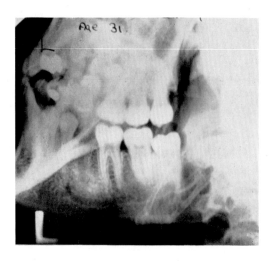

Fig. 548.—Eruption cyst around the crown of |8.

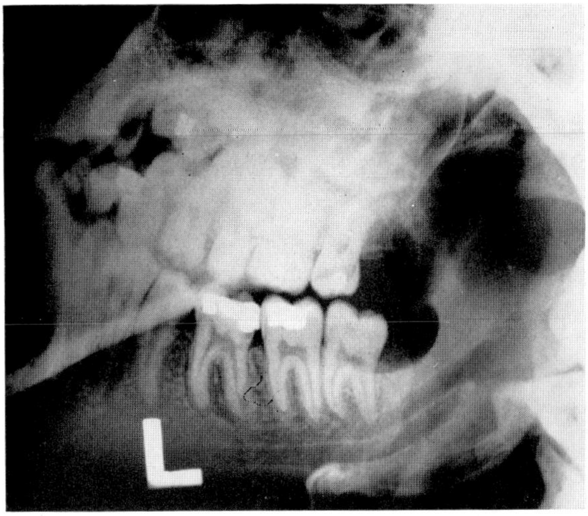

Fig. 549.—Eruption cyst lateral to the partially erupted crown of |8 and extending upwards along the lower part of the anterior border of the ascending ramus.

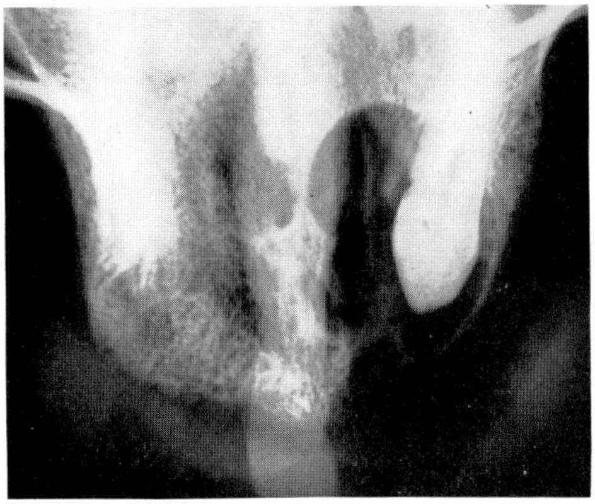

Fig. 550.—Mesial dentigerous cyst associated with proximal half of unerupted |3.

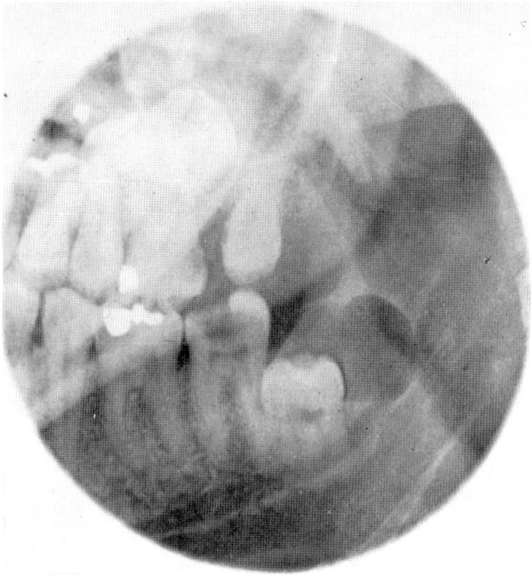

Fig. 551.—Unerupted |8 with lateral dentigerous cyst.

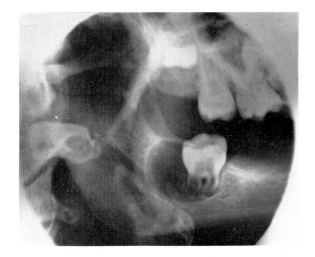

Fig. 552.—8| almost fully erupted with associated lateral dentigerous cyst.

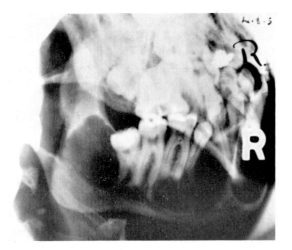

Fig. 553.—Partially erupted 8| with lateral dentigerous cyst extending half-way up the ascending ramus.

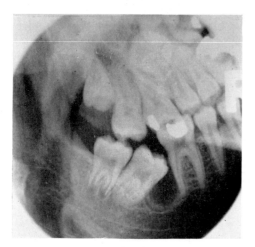

Fig. 554.—Partially erupted 7| with mesial dentigerous cyst.

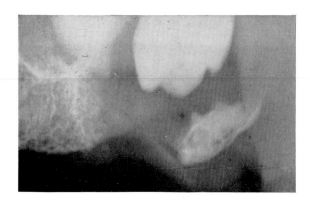

Fig. 555.—Unerupted |8 with dentigerous cyst carrying bony flake of the tuberosity incorporated in its wall.

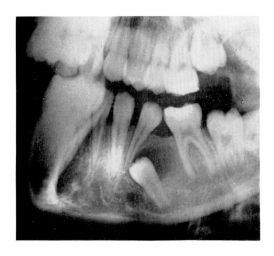

Fig. 556.—Unerupted |5 displaced down towards the inferior dental canal, with dentigerous cyst associated with crown only.

Fig. 557.—Unerupted |6 with apices almost penetrating the lower border of the mandible, with dentigerous cyst around the crown only. |7 unerupted with follicular eruption cyst.

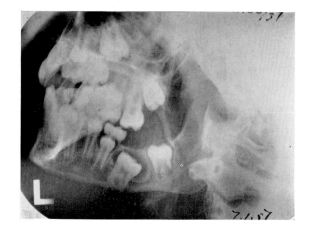

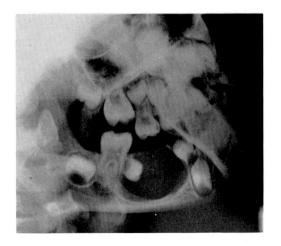

Fig. 558.—Unerupted $\overline{5|}$ completely enclosed in a large dentigerous cyst. The unerupted tooth is lying in the horizontal axis of the mandible with its distal end against the $\overline{6|}$. $\overline{4|}$ is unerupted and displaced mesially and above the unerupted $\overline{3|}$.

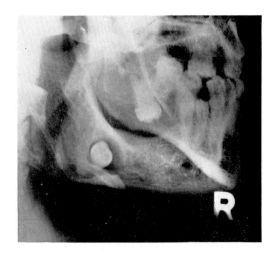

Fig. 559.—$\overline{8|}$ unerupted and deeply situated near the angle of the mandible. It is completely enclosed in a dentigerous cyst. The patient is 34 years of age and only the crown of the unerupted $\overline{8|}$ is formed.

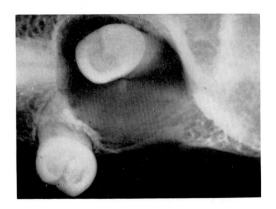

Fig. 560.—Unerupted $|\underline{5}$ lying beneath the floor of the left antrum in a dentigerous cyst. The distal part of the unerupted $|\underline{3}$ can be seen above the erupted $|\underline{4}$ and in contact with the cyst wall.

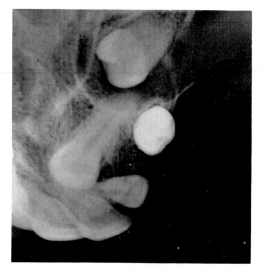

Fig. 561.—Same patient as in *Fig.* 560. Occlusal view of the unerupted |5 and the dentigerous cyst.

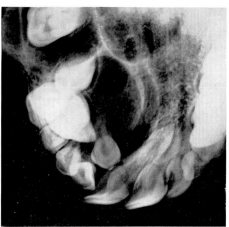

Fig. 562.—Occlusal view showing a dentigerous cyst at the anterior part of the palate. 5432| are unerupted.

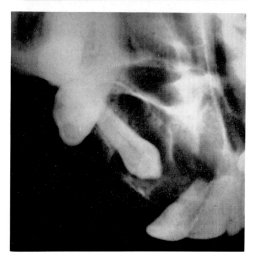

Fig. 563.—Unerupted 3| associated with a large multilocular dentigerous cyst extending across the midline of the palate.

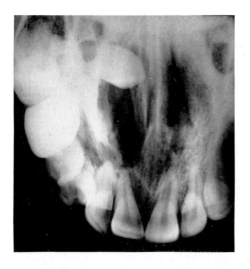

Fig. 564.—The dentigerous cyst is situated in the long axis of the palate, confined to its own half, and displacing posteriorly the unerupted 3|.

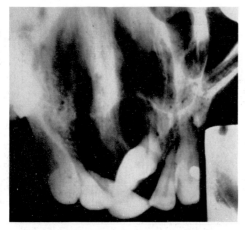

Fig. 565.—Dentigerous cyst around the unerupted |1. The cyst has extended beyond the midline of the palate.

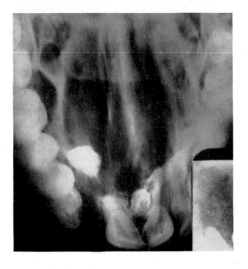

Fig. 566.—Dentigerous cyst associated with an unerupted supernumerary tooth in the 2| region. There is another unerupted supernumerary tooth in the upper central incisor region.

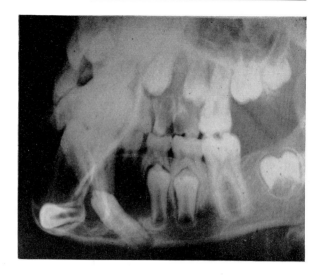

Fig. 567.—The two mandibular canines are unerupted, situated at the lower border of the mandible. There is a dentigerous cyst around the lower left unerupted canine.

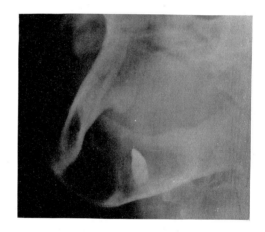

Fig. 568.—Patient, aged 61 years, with history extending over ten years of a progressive swelling in the anterior part of the lower jaw. Increasing pain during the last six months.

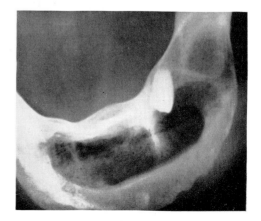

Fig. 569.—Occlusal view of *Fig.* 568. Unerupted |3̄ in large multilocular dentigerous cyst with grossly thickened walls. Much pus was evacuated at operation.

17

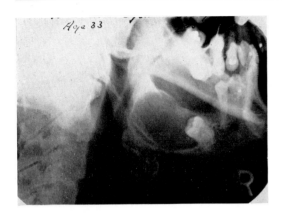

Fig. 570.—Unerupted 6̄| with denti-gerous cyst extending up the ramus. There is backward and downward displacement of the inferior dental canal.

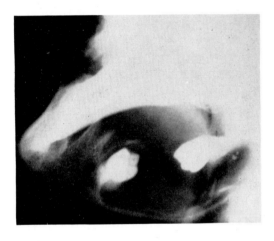

Fig. 571.—Unerupted |6̄ with large dentigerous cyst extending upwards along the ascending ramus and dis-placing the unerupted |8̄.

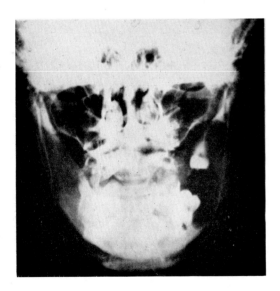

Fig. 572.—Same patient as in *Fig.* 571. Postero-anterior view showing the involvement of the ramus and the superficial position of the unerupted |8̄.

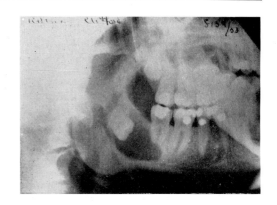

Fig. 573.—Unerupted $\overline{8|}$ enclosed in a dentigerous cyst. The cyst in its growth is carrying the unerupted $\overline{8|}$ up the ramus.

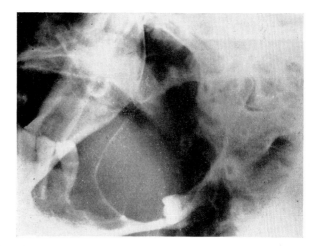

Figs. 574, 575.—Unerupted $\overline{|8}$ displaced to the lower border of the mandible at the angle, with an associated dentigerous cyst involving the whole of the ascending ramus.

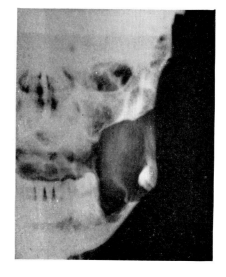

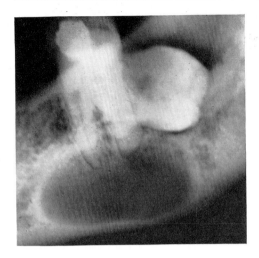

Fig. 576.—Unerupted $\overline{8}$ with a biloculated dentigerous cyst.

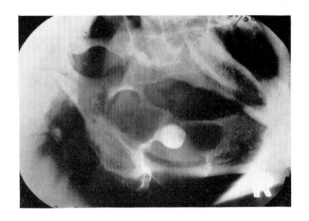

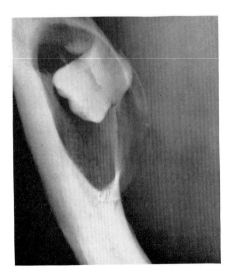

Figs. 577, 578.—Unerupted $\overline{8}|$ surrounded by a multilocular dentigerous cyst, and involving the molar region and ascending ramus.

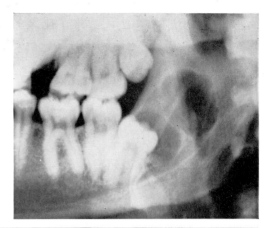

Fig. 579.—Unerupted 8 with multi-locular dentigerous cyst extending up to the mandibular notch.

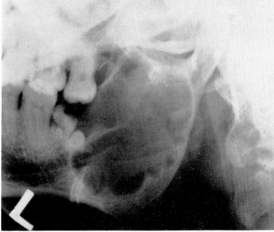

Fig. 580.—Unerupted 8 and rudimentary supernumerary associated with a large multilocular dentigerous cyst, involving the whole of the ascending ramus.

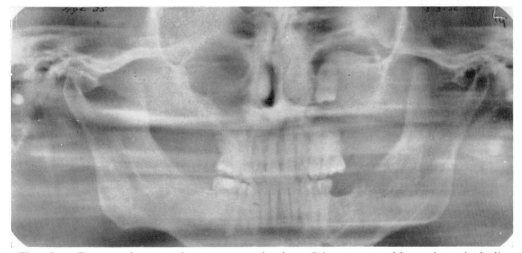

Fig. 581.—Rotograph presenting a panoramic view of the upper and lower jaws, including both temporomandibular joints. A large dentigerous cyst carrying an unerupted 8 is occupying almost the whole of the left sinus cavity.

Periodontal or Radicular Cysts

THE periodontal cyst is of chronic low-grade infective origin. It is the commonest cyst in the jaws and is found in connexion with an infected tooth, root, or socket. The age incidence is from 10 years to late life, and the cyst may be situated in any part of either jaw, in both jaws simultaneously, or multiple in the same jaw. Occasionally the cyst forms laterally at the side of the distal end of the root.

The cyst develops from an epitheliated granuloma which has formed at the apex of a tooth. The internal structure of the granuloma disintegrates, vacuolates, and leaves a central cavity surrounded by a fibrous capsule lined with epithelium.

Periodontal cysts vary considerably in size, enlarging by extension and expansion. Their size and shape are dependent upon the resistance offered by the immediate tissues.

If slow growing, a periodontal cyst retains its circular outline with an intact cortical wall. The more rapid the growth, the poorer the outline of the cyst, coincident with resorption of the surrounding bone.

The cyst may extend axially along the length of the mandible and assume an elongated shape. In the maxilla, the cyst may encroach upon and enter the nasal fossa or antrum. In its enlargement, the cyst may deflect or rotate standing teeth or displace such structures as the inferior dental canal, the median suture, or the posterior palatine foramen.

Radiographically, a periodontal cyst is seen as a circular translucent black area enclosed by a sharply-defined white radio-opaque thin cortical wall. This wall is continuous with the lamina dura of the socket, except in the case of the residual cyst which lies below the alveolar margin. The mouth of the tooth socket is bridged over by new bone formation.

The root and apices of the tooth from which the cyst arises need not necessarily show signs of erosion or resorption, although the tooth itself may be root-filled. The tooth usually shows evidence of caries of the crown and signs of pulpitis.

Secondary infection of a periodontal cyst is quite a common occurrence, and when suppuration takes place within the cyst, the black translucent area becomes grey and hazy, and the cortical wall ill-defined and sometimes broken.

Some of these cysts become multiloculated and present a scalloped cortical contour. They are erroneously described as adamantinomas.

Occasionally, isolated periodontal cysts are found in edentulous areas of the jaws. These are probably residual periodontal cysts where the teeth have been extracted without the presence of a cyst being suspected or recognized. It may be impossible to distinguish them from primordial cysts.

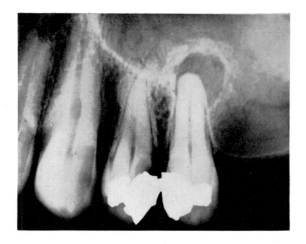

Fig. 582.—Apical granuloma or small periodontal cyst, discovered during routine X-ray examination. Hazy translucency in an encapsulated circular area. The outer cortical wall is continuous with the lamina dura of the |5. The lesion is invaginating the floor of the antrum.

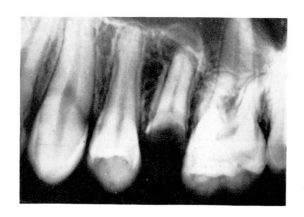

Fig. 583.—Small periodontal cyst in connexion with root |5 lying below the floor of the left antrum.

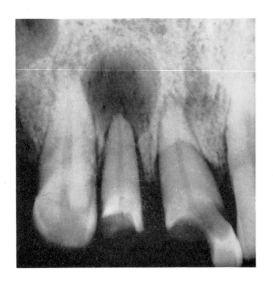

Fig. 584.—2| periodontal cyst with ill-defined outer cortical wall. The inner area shows numerous small black spots in a hazy opacity—superimposed infection.

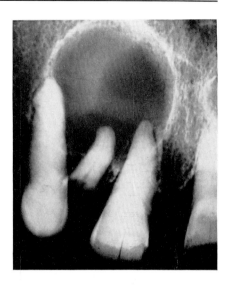

Fig. 585.—2| periodontal cyst found in a patient, aged 72 years. History of recurrent swelling for at least 15 years. The thickened cortical wall may be due to long-standing osteoblastic reaction. Much purulent matter was evacuated when root was extracted.

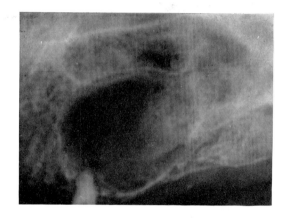

Fig. 586.—|5 root with associated periodontal cyst. The continuity of the cortical wall with the socket of the root differentiates it from a loculus of the antrum.

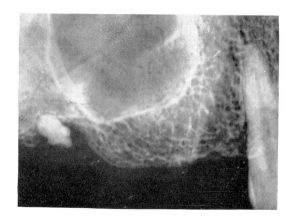

Fig. 587.—The radiolucent area in 654| region is *not* a periodontal cyst. The cortical wall is not continuous with the socket of the retained 6| root, and the internal translucent area contains the image of the channel carrying the antral vessels.

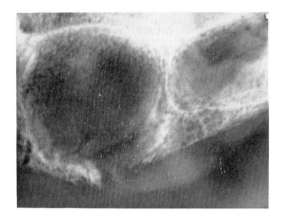

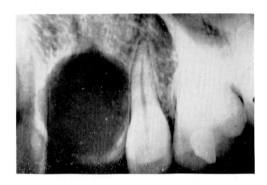

Fig. 588.—The mesial translucent area in the |345 region is a periodontal cyst with its outer cortical wall continuous with the empty |4 socket. The distal area in the |678 region is the shadow of the antrum and has no connexion with any tooth, root, or socket. It is oval in shape and not circular.

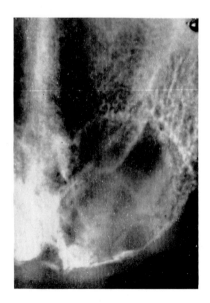

Fig. 589.—Residual periodontal cyst in |34 region. The teeth were removed some years previously without a radiographic examination, and with no knowledge of the existence of an underlying cyst.

Fig. 590.—Residual periodontal cyst in |123 region. Early signs of expansion of the cyst wall bucally, and extension into the nasal fossa.

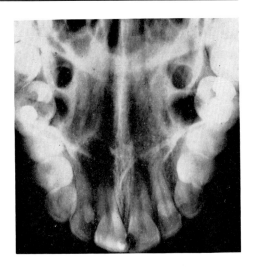

Fig. 591.—Occlusal view of the upper jaw. ı| region, periodontal cyst; |ı region, periapical abscess. In the first molar regions, the images of anterior loculi of the antra are seen bilaterally, with the nasolacrimal foramina posteriorly.

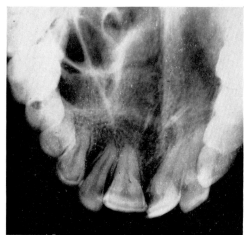

Fig. 592.—Occlusal view showing a periodontal cyst extending internally into the hard palate from 5| and displacing the nasolacrimal foramen towards the midline.

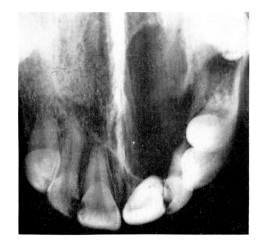

Fig. 593.—Occlusal view depicting a periodontal cyst involving the hard palate on one side and extending backwards longitudinally. It has not crossed the midline.

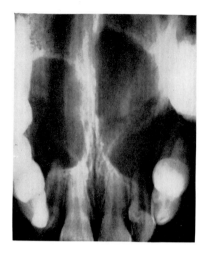

Fig. 594.—Occlusal view of bilateral periodontal cysts separated and limited by the median suture of the maxilla.

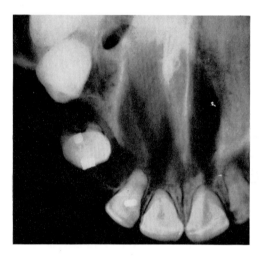

Fig. 595.—Occlusal view of a unilateral periodontal cyst crossing the midline and expanding the outer wall of the maxilla.

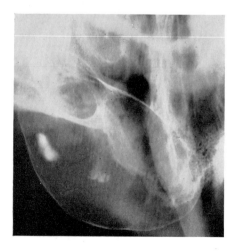

Fig. 596.—Large unilateral distended periodontal cyst in association with retained roots 543|. Gross expansion of the outer wall of the maxilla.

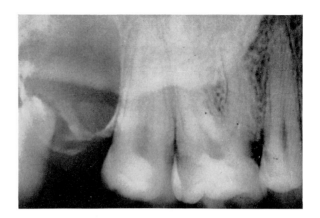

Fig. 597.—Dental cyst incorporated in the tuberosity of the maxilla, with overlying shadow of the coronoid process.

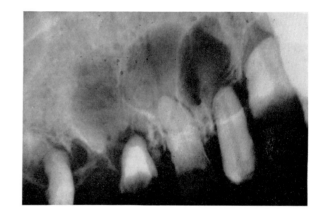

Fig. 598.—Multiple periodontal cysts in connexion with roots 54321|.

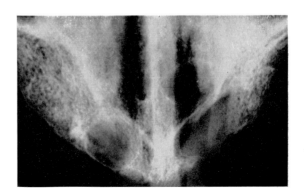

Fig. 599.—Multiple periodontal cysts in an edentulous upper jaw in 21|123 region.

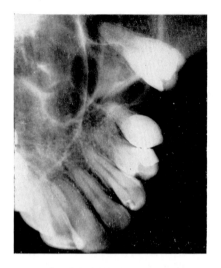

Fig. 600.—Occlusal view depicting a circumscribed translucent area in the |6 region requiring differentiation between a loculus of the left antrum or a residual periodontal cyst.

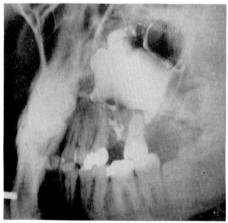

Fig. 601.—Lateral oblique view of *Fig.* 600, showing the introduction of lipiodol into the cavity by injection through the empty socket of |6. The fully filled hollow adopts the normal quadrilateral outline with rounded corners of the maxillary antrum.

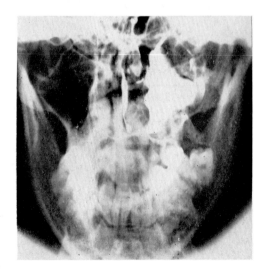

Fig. 602.—Postero-anterior view of *Figs.* 600, 601. The overflow of the contrast medium into the nasal fossa through the ostium is conclusive proof that the translucent area seen in *Fig.* 600 is the shadow of the antrum and not that of a periodontal cyst.

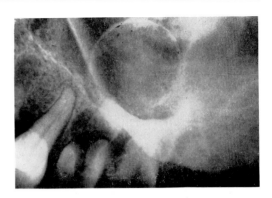

Fig. 603.—Intra-oral view, showing a periodontal cyst arising from roots |67 and entering the left maxillary sinus.

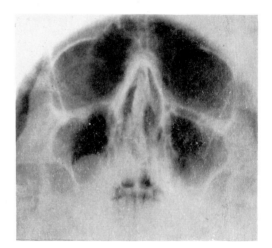

Figs. 604, 605.—Postero-anterior view of two different patients depicting suppurating periodontal cysts in the right and left antra respectively. The upper convex outline of the cysts distinguishes them from empyemas which present a horizontal fluid level.

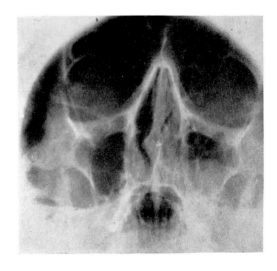

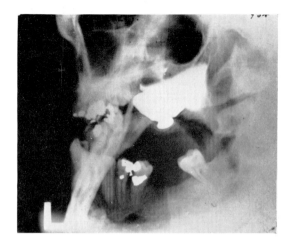

Fig. 606.—Lipiodol injection into a periodontal cyst. The radiolucent shadow of the left antrum is seen above it.

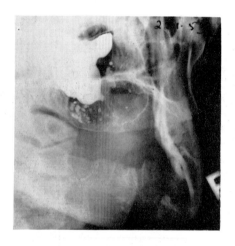

Fig. 607.—Lipiodol introduced into the right antrum and presenting the normal outline of the sinus. Below it is the translucent area of a periodontal cyst.

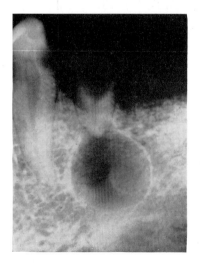

Fig. 608.—A periodontal cyst in connexion with a retained root $\overline{|5}$, and showing the continuity of the outer cortical wall of the cyst with the lamina dura of the socket.

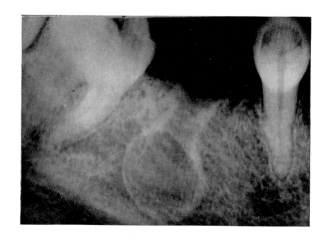

Fig. 609.—$\overline{5|}$ region. An un-suspected periodontal cyst found during an all-round routine X-ray examination.

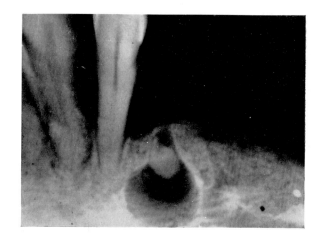

Fig. 610.—A periodontal cyst in $\overline{|4}$ region. The retained root has fallen into the cyst.

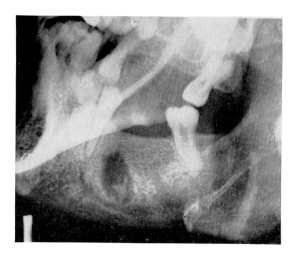

Fig. 611.—Routine X-ray examin-ation revealed the presence of a root fragment in a translucent area. At operation, the root was removed and a pathological examination identi-fied the lesion as a periodontal cyst, into which the root had fallen and over which new bone had formed and created a residual cyst.

18

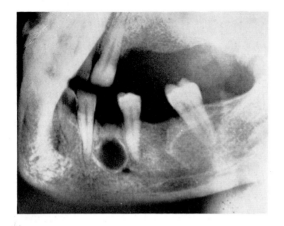

Fig. 612.—Extra-oral view of a periodontal cyst with retained root $\overline{|4}$. The cortical cyst wall is in close approximation to the mental foramen.

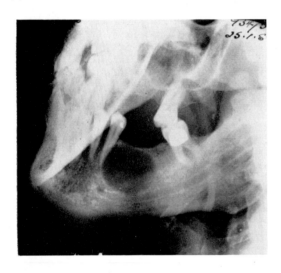

Fig. 613.—Extra-oral view of a residual dental cyst in the mandibular first molar region, lying above the inferior dental canal.

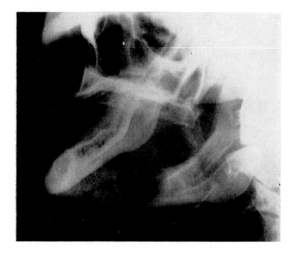

Fig. 614.—Extra-oral view of an expanding periodontal cyst depressing and displacing the proximal part of the inferior dental canal.

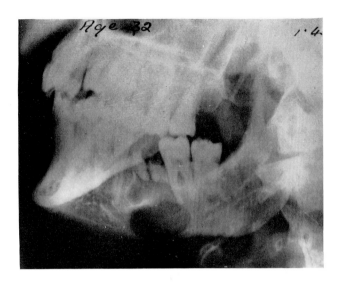

Fig. 615.—Multilocular peri-odontal cyst in connexion with roots |6̄. The anterior part of the inferior dental canal is displaced downwards towards the lower border of the man-dible.

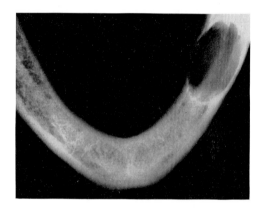

Fig. 616.—Occlusal view of a residual periodontal cyst lying in the long axis of the mandible between the inner and outer walls of the lower jaw.

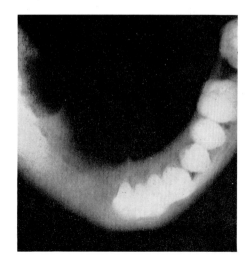

Fig. 617.—Occlusal view of a peri-odontal cyst lying on the lingual aspect of the mandible.

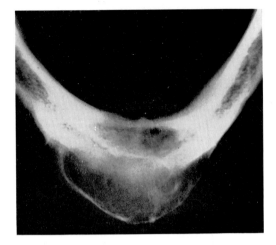

Fig. 618.—Occlusal view of a peri-odontal cyst lying on the buccal aspect of the mandible at the symphysis menti.

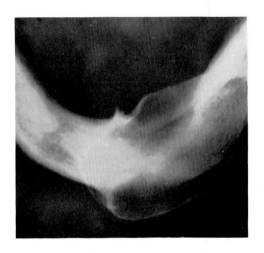

Fig. 619.—The periodontal cyst situated in the $\overline{1234}$ region is multiloculated.

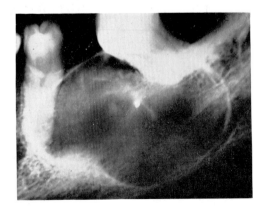

Fig. 620.—The periodontal cyst arising in the $\overline{6}$ region is grossly distended. The end-on view presents a radiographic illusion of overlapping of the roots of $\overline{5}$ and $\overline{7}$.

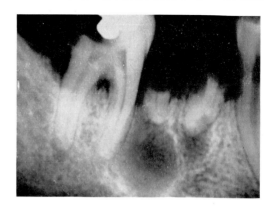

Fig. 621.—Two separate periodontal cysts in connexion with the two separate retained roots of 6̅|.

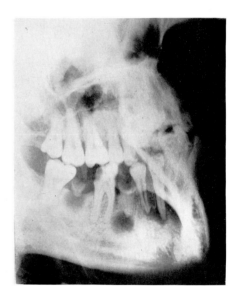

Fig. 622.—Two separate small periodontal cysts associated with roots 7̅| and 5̅|.

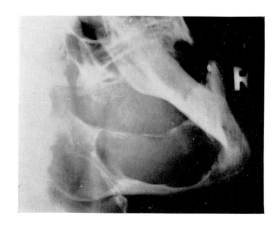

Fig. 623.—Large periodontal cyst involving the whole of the horizontal body of the mandible.

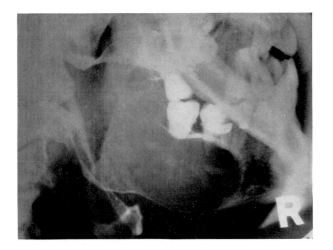

Fig. 624.—Large periodontal cyst involving the distal half of the mandible, the angle of the jaw, and all of the ascending ramus, including the coronoid process, the mandibular notch, and the base of the condylar process.

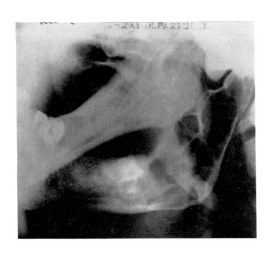

Fig. 625.—Multilocular periodontal cyst involving the whole of the ascending ramus.

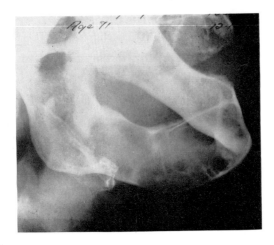

Fig. 626.—Extra-oral view of a large multilocular periodontal cyst occupying the body of the mandible and simulating an ameloblastoma.

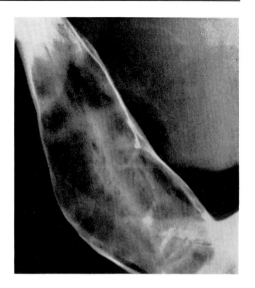

Fig. 627.—Occlusal view of *Fig.* 626. The histopathological report confirmed that the lesion was a periodontal cyst.

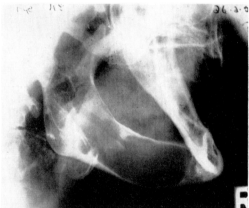

Fig. 628.—Extra-oral view of an extensive periodontal cyst occupying the whole of the right mandible from symphysis menti to the mandibular notch.

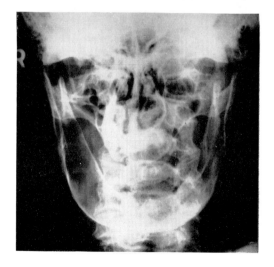

Fig. 629.—Postero-anterior view of *Fig.* 628. The expansion of the mandible is not grossly manifest.

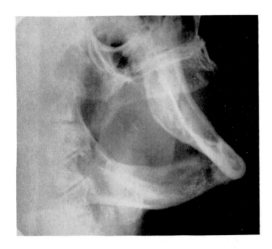

Figs. 630, 631.—The same patient as in *Figs.* 628, 629, one year later after operation. Both views show almost complete bone regeneration.

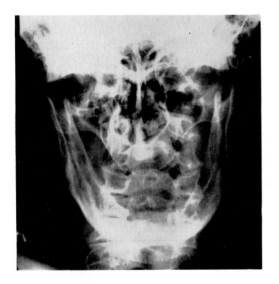

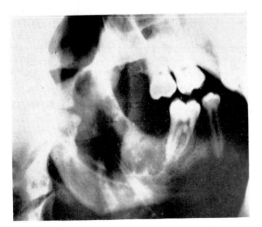

Fig. 632.—Large multilocular periodontal cyst extending from the right lower third molar region to the mandibular notch and coronoid process.

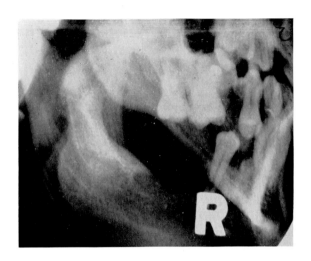

Fig. 633.—Same patient as in *Fig.* 632. Apparent complete removal of the multilocular cyst eighteen months previously with no signs of any recurrence.

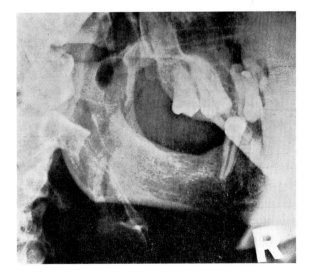

Fig. 634.—Two years exactly after removal of the cyst shown in *Fig.* 632. Recurring cyst involving the coronoid process and the upper part of the right ascending ramus anterior to the inferior dental canal.

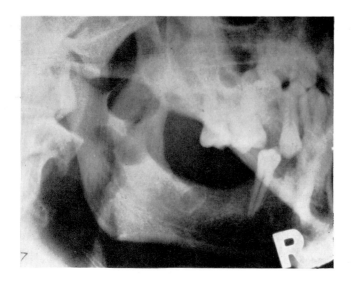

Fig. 635.—Sixteen months after the radiograph shown in *Fig.* 634 additional confluent cystic lesions are seen in the upper part of the ascending ramus. A solitary cyst has developed in the molar region 8̄|.

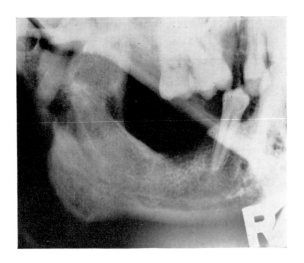

Fig. 636.—Twenty-seven months after the removal of the cysts seen in *Fig.* 635. Apparent progressive bone regeneration with no signs of cystic formation.

Traumatic Cysts

Hæmorrhagic Cysts.—Hæmorrhagic cysts are rare lesions which are found more commonly in the mandible. The actual cause is not well understood, although there is an associated history of an external injury, in many cases, some years previously. These cysts have been described as occurring chiefly in young people.

The hæmorrhagic cyst is usually asymptomatic and found during a routine radiographic examination.

The radiograph shows a solitary radiolucent area, more often below the roots of the teeth in the mandible in the premolar-molar region, but it may extend into the ramus. The contour is irregular and may be devoid of the sharp white limiting line seen in a periodontal cyst.

The cystic condition is not connected with any root or tooth; it may extend along the roots and even displace them, but the roots are not involved. The radiolucent area rarely reaches the alveolar margin. Because of the low internal fluid pressure, the hæmorrhagic cyst rarely shows signs of expansion.

In the older patient these lesions are alluded to as 'latent hæmorrhagic bone cysts', and are distinguished by a thick cortex surrounding the hæmorrhagic cavity.

Clinically, the teeth overlying the hæmorrhagic cyst are vital, and the ultimate diagnosis can be made only in the histopathological department. The enveloping fibrous sac is devoid of epithelium and may contain shreds of friable dark red tissue, blood-stained fluid, or yellow xanthomatous cholesterol ester cells. The hæmorrhagic cyst is prone to secondary infection.

Occasionally, a radiograph of a periapical abscess in the upper incisor region reveals an open apex of the root without any resorption. The tooth is fully developed and vital before the apex generally closes; there is a history of trauma during the period of 10–12 years of age.

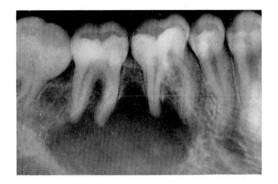

Fig. 637.—Radiolucent area in $\overline{76|}$ region below the roots. Irregular contour with no signs of a cortical wall. The roots appear to be invaginating the hæmorrhagic cyst.

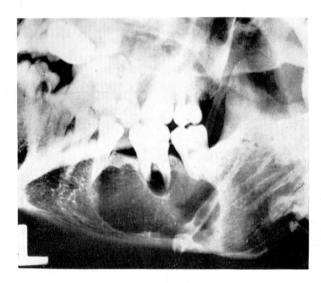

Fig. 638.—Latent hæmorrhagic cyst in $|\overline{5678}$ region. The contour is clear cut but there is no defined cortical wall. The bone trabeculations within the image of the cyst are images of the buccal and lingual walls of the mandible.

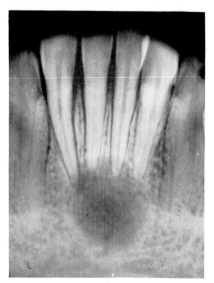

Fig. 639.—Hæmorrhagic cyst in the $\overline{1|1}$ region. This is a site of predilection and an area prone to trauma. The radiolucent area is ill-defined and has not reached the alveolar margin. All the incisor teeth are vital.

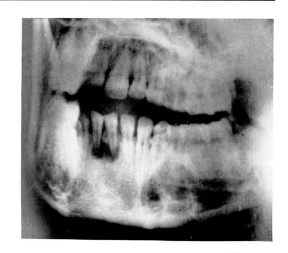

Fig. 640.—Hæmorrhagic cyst in the lower central incisor region. At operation, black stained fluid was evacuated, and the histopathological examination stated that the fibrous sac was devoid of epithelium.

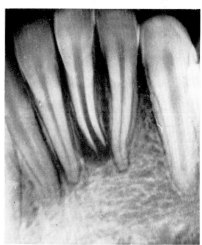

Fig. 641.—|1̄ small apical hæmorrhagic cyst with open apex in a patient aged 18 years, discovered during routine radiographic examination. History of a blow on the chin when 8 years old.

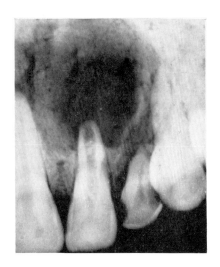

Fig. 642.—|2 traumatic hæmorrhagic cyst in patient aged 21 years. Apex open, no resorption of the root. Traumatic history at age of 11 years.

Non-odontogenic Cysts

NON-ODONTOGENIC cysts have no connexion with the teeth. They fall into two groups, fissural and incisive canal cysts.

1. Fissural Cysts are formed from epithelial cells enclaved in the line of fusion of various embryonic processes of the face.

 a. *Median Cysts* are found mainly in the line of the median fissure of the maxilla.

   The alveolar type are centrally placed between the roots of the central incisors. The teeth are rarely pressed apart, and the median cysts adapt themselves to an elliptical shape. In the edentulous patient, the cyst tends to become more circular.

   The palatal type of median cyst lies farther back in the posterior part of the palate.

 b. *Globulomaxillary Cysts* form at the junction of the premaxilla and maxillary processes in the alveolar bone. They are located between the upper lateral incisor and canine teeth, and cause them to diverge. They may grow to a large size and extend posteriorly in the palate.

2. Incisive Canal Cysts are varieties of nasopalatine cysts, and are located in the alveolar process of the maxilla. The cysts are usually situated in the midline, but may extend symmetrically or unilaterally. Occasionally, two distinct cysts may be seen, separate or fused, and the latter present a heart-shaped appearance.

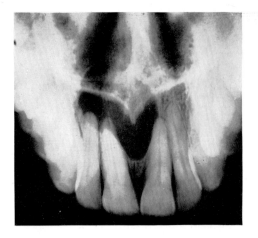

Fig. 643.—Alveolar midline cyst situated in the anterior part of the median fissure of the maxilla, between the roots of the upper central incisors. The distal halves of the teeth are being pushed apart.

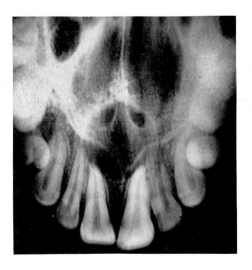

Fig. 644.—Alveolar median cyst lying just posterior to the roots of the upper central incisors, which are not displaced. The contour is well defined and circular in shape.

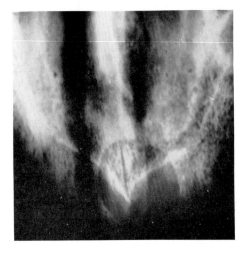

Fig. 645.—Alveolar median cyst in an edentulous maxilla, found on routine radiographic examination. It simulates a residual periodontal cyst.

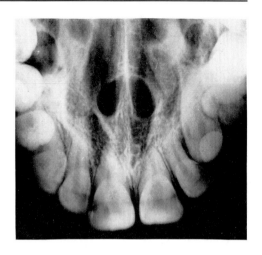

Fig. 646.—Palatal median cyst, lying farther back in the hard palate.

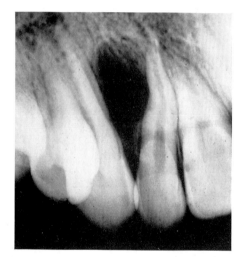

Fig. 647.—Globulomaxillary cyst at the junction of the right premaxilla and maxillary process. It is pear shaped and causing divarication of the lateral incisor and canine teeth.

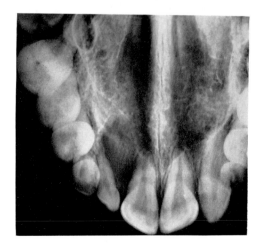

Fig. 648.—Globulomaxillary cyst in the 3̲2̲| region with retained c̲b̲| and absent 3̲2̲|. The cyst is extending backwards into the hard palate.

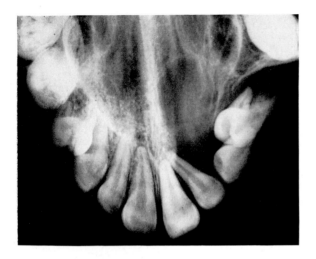

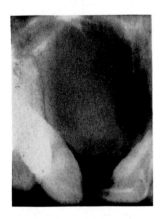

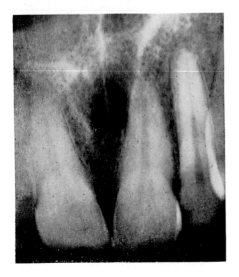

Fig. 649.—Globulomaxillary cyst easily mistaken for a residual periodontal cyst. The cyst wall was a thick fibrous structure, firmly attached to the surrounding bone. The inner lining was ciliated epithelium.

Fig. 650.—Globulomaxillary cyst in the 3̲2̲| region. Three days' history of an acute painful swelling from which was evacuated a copious amount of pus. Had been identified many years previously as a globulomaxillary cyst.

Fig. 651.—Incisive canal cyst located in the alveolar process of the mandible in the midline, between the apices of 1̲|1̲.

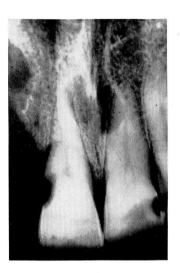

Fig. 652.—Two distinct incisive canal cysts, which are fused, presenting a heart-shaped appearance. The radiograph gives the illusion of the cysts overlying the apices of 1|1.

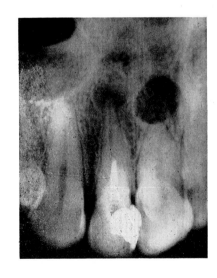

Fig. 653.—Incisive canal cyst in the 1| region. Periapical granuloma associated with 2|.

II.—Tumours of the Jaws and Mouth

　　1. Odontogenic tumours.

　　2. Osteogenic tumours.

　　3. Intra-osseous or central tumours.

　　4. Soft-tissue tumours.

　　5. Systemic diseases.

Tumours of the Jaws and Mouth

TUMOURS of the jaws and mouth may be classified as:—

1. Odontogenic tumours.
2. Osteogenic tumours.
3. Central intra-osseous tumours.
4. Soft-tissue tumours of the mouth.

The diagnosis of tumours of the jaws is more definite to-day with the employment of modern methods of radiographic examination. Much information is furnished thereby, but radiography should not be relied upon to the exclusion of other diagnostic methods.

Certain tumours disclose characteristic radiographic features, and the findings revealed by the X rays are dependent upon:—

1. Location of the Tumour.—Tumours of bone have sites of predilection.

2. Mode of Growth.—A solitary tumour may be encapsulated and its growth cause expansion of the bone without destruction. This may produce a unilateral asymmetry. Multiple growths of the jaw may be associated with a general skeletal distribution and show distinct symmetry. Metastatic tumours grow from the centre and invade the surrounding tissue.

3. Bone Production.—Tumours growing from the central part of a main bone may stimulate the surrounding osseous tissue to produce irregular new bone formation. If the tumour is located at the periphery of the bone it is important to note whether the new bone formation is deposited parallel or at right angles to the cortex.

4. Bone Destruction.—A malignant growth destroys bone by progressive infiltration. A benign neoplasm may produce erosion of the bone purely by pressure atrophy.

In some cases, osteolytic reaction may result in resorption and replacement of bone simultaneously.

Odontogenic Tumours

ODONTOGENIC tumours are composed of part or all of the tissues of the dental follicle. Some produce calcified tooth substances and are called hard or calcified odontomes. These have been described on p. 92. When there is complete absence of calcium within these odontomes they are classified as soft odontomes.

The only soft odontomes which present some distinguishable radiographic features are the ameloblastomas and fibromas, but these are by no means absolute.

Ameloblastomas are formed principally from the cells of the enamel organ, but do not contain any enamel formation. They are usually discovered and identified during the third decade of life, although their formation must have begun at a much earlier stage. Cases have been detected as late as 75 years of age.

The tumours are markedly slow in their growth and, while considered essentially benign in character, nevertheless they must be regarded as potentially local malignant neoplasms.

Ameloblastomas are mainly central tumours and are found in both jaws, more commonly in the premolar and molar regions of the mandible, and particularly in the ramus. In the upper jaw they may extend into the maxillary antrum, the orbit, and the nasopharynx.

Radiographically, there are no special characteristics by which these entities may be recognized and differentiated from similar lesions. There are, however, two definite types of ameloblastomas:—

1. *The monocystic ameloblastoma*, the less common variety, is a solid, soft-tissue growth and allows the X rays to pass through it and cast a hazy translucent shadow on the radiograph. The outline is irregular, lobulated, and often notched, and its cortical wall is not continuous with the lamina dura of a tooth. The roots of any nearby teeth may be completely denuded of any supporting structure. Teeth or tooth remnants may be found within the lesion, and adjoining teeth are rarely displaced. There may be a number of small accessory cyst-like shadows at the periphery of the tumour.

2. *The polycystic ameloblastoma* resembles a multilocular cyst with a great variation in the size and shape of the numerous cavities within the lesion. Some of the tumours show a honeycomb pattern. In this type, the teeth may be displaced or tilted and the roots resorbed.

Other soft odontomes, such as odontogenic myxomas and fibromas, are benign in character and cast no definite images. The only clue as to their nature is a biopsy examination.

Odontogenic Fibromas.—These are solitary central tumours of the jaw, developing at the apex of a tooth. Their association with the roots of a tooth is in conformity with its seat of origin from the mesenchymal portion of the tooth germ.

The tumour is slow growing, but may develop to a large size and cause expansion of the bone. It may be mistaken for a granuloma or periodontal cyst.

The X-ray appearance of this benign growth is that of a cystic condition in connexion with the roots of a tooth. It has a well-defined margin and is most often associated with the lower molar teeth. The translucent shadow may exhibit small radio-opaque particles within its midst.

The growth may change its character and become malignant. In such circumstances, the outer peripheral limit loses its sharp demarcation and extends irregularly into the immediate tissues.

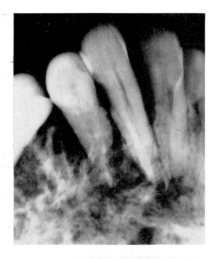

Fig. 654.—Ameloblastoma. $\overline{65432}|$ region shows a large area of bone destruction, simulating osteomyelitis or metastatic carcinoma. The appearance is not typical of an ameloblastoma. The denudation of the roots of the teeth, which are not displaced or tilted, is characteristic of the presence of a tumour.

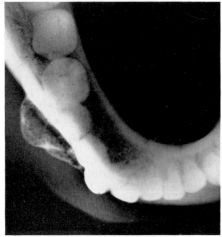

Fig. 655.—Ameloblastoma. This occlusal view of *Fig.* 654 dismisses the possibility of osteomyelitis. It suggests a new growth formation of a multilocular type producing expansion of the outer wall of the mandible.

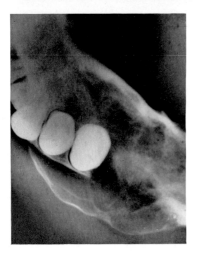

Fig. 656.—Ameloblastoma. This radiograph of an ameloblastoma shows a multilocular condition associated with a lesion which has replaced the normal bone trabeculation. No sign of new bone formation.

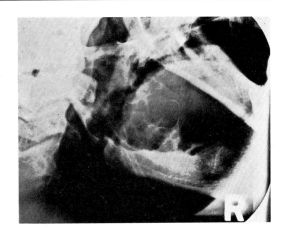

Fig. 657.—Polycystic ameloblastoma in a male, aged 31 years. A small cyst in the 8| region was removed eight years previously but not examined histologically. The present lesion is associated with a swelling of about three months' duration.

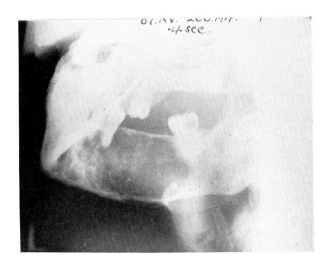

Fig. 658.—Ameloblastoma, solid type. |34567 region depicts loss of bone trabeculation, no cystic formation, and no alveolar or lower border bone expansion.

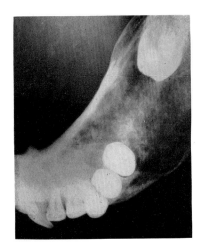

Fig. 659.—Ameloblastoma. Occlusal view of *Fig.* 658 shows the existence of a soft-tissue formation with bone infiltration and expansion.

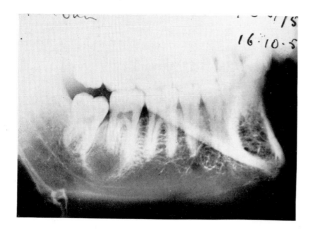

Fig. 660.—Odontogenic fibroma. A localized circular area below the $\overline{7|}$ in close proximity to the inferior dental canal. It simulates an apical abscess or epitheliated granuloma, but there is no sign of any caries in the tooth.

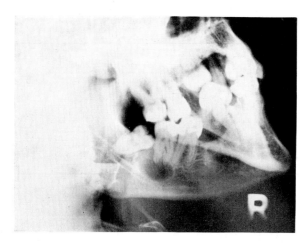

Fig. 661.—Odontogenic fibroma. A pseudocystic appearance overlying the apices of $\overline{7|}$ in the cancellous part of the mandible. It has a well-defined cortical wall. The fact that it is oval in shape and that the cortical wall is not continuous with the lamina dura of the socket wall of the $\overline{7|}$ contraindicates a periodontal cyst.

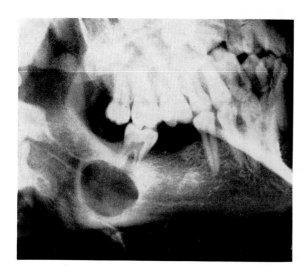

Fig. 662.—Odontogenic fibroma. The large radiolucent area overlies the inferior dental canal at the angle of the right mandible and reaches almost to the lower border of the mandible. Its sharply cut margin suggests a punched-out lesion. The ill-defined, semi-opaque bodies with the radiolucent area are cementicles which are characteristic of this odontogenic formation.

Osteogenic Tumours

OSTEOGENIC tumours arise from bone cells or bone-forming tissues and occur at any stage of adult life. They are commonly met with in or about the jaws and may interfere with the true seating of a denture. They can be benign or malignant in character.

Benign Osteogenic Tumours.—

1. *Dysostoses*.—These are overgrowths or deposits of new bone and not true tumours, and are seen as localized or diffuse formations.

   a. *Exostosis* is a localized, circumscribed overgrowth of bone of common occurrence, forming along the alveolar margin or from the walls of the mandible or maxilla. It may be single or multiple and frequently found at the insertion of muscles and tendons, or at the junction of two bones. There is often an associated history of trauma or inflammatory stimulation, such as an ill-fitting denture.

   On the radiograph the exostosis is seen either as a pointed, nodular, tuberous, or globular cancellated outgrowth of bone. It is continuous with the main bone and may be sessile or pedunculated.

   Exostotic enlargement of the genial tubercles is not uncommon. Torus palatinus and torus mandibularis are two specialized forms. The former occurs in the midline of the hard palate, in its posterior part, as a dense, flat, or nodular sessile growth, often lobulated. Torus mandibularis appears as bilateral, round protuberances arising from the lingual surface of the mandible, in the premolar region. The outgrowths may fuse to form a horizontal shelf in the floor of the mouth and interfere with the free movement of the tongue.

   b. *Enostosis* is a localized overgrowth of bone arising from the spongiosa of the jaws, and is akin to an endosteal osteoma. It is commonly found in the premolar and molar regions of the mandible and is seen on the radiograph as a circumscribed, dense, opaque structure, often with a bursa-like capsule.

   c. *Hyperostosis* is a diffuse overgrowth of part or the whole of a bone, usually confined to one side of the face. The commonest areas are the upper molar region and maxillary tuberosity and the condylar process and angle of the mandible.

   Trauma and inflammatory conditions appear to play important parts as exciting causes.

   Multiple hyperostoses are seen in the skull in such systemic diseases as Paget's disease, acromegaly, and leontiasis ossea. Radiographically, the area involved exhibits a diffuse radio-opaque mass with fine, closely knit uniform bone network. The cortex may be expanded, the teeth displaced, and normal anatomical structures, such as the maxillary sinus and inferior dental canal, pushed from their normal siting.

2. *Osteomas*.—These tumours arise from retained embryonic cartilage cells, from the periosteum, and from established bone. They are benign tumours of slow progressive growth and many appear traumatic in origin. They are found both at the periphery and in the central part of the bone.

Two different types can be distinguished on the radiograph:—

    a. Osteoma durum or eburnum: This is seen as an opaque, dense, pedunculated, or sessile mass, varying in size from that of a pea to a table-tennis ball. This form may grow so large as to involve half of the face. The common sites are the molar region in the maxilla and the premolar area and lower border in the mandible. Osteomas are frequently found arising from the bony walls of the frontal and maxillary sinuses.

    b. Osteoma spongiosum: This rare type of bone tumour is found mainly in the mandible. It is depicted as a circumscribed area, encompassed by an opaque ring of new bone formation, and, in its centre, spongiosa with widened bone network and translucent areas.

Both types of osteoma may grow to a very large size and produce gross facial disfigurement. When found inside the mouth, the tumour interferes with speech, mastication, and swallowing. Cases of multiple osteomas are not infrequent.

    3. *Chondromas*.—These rare tumours form from embryonic cartilage cells and appear at an early age as outgrowths from the bone surface. Central chondromas have been reported.

The usual sites are the upper central region, the coronoid and condylar processes, and the symphysis menti. The tumour is benign, slow growing, and usually encapsulated. If allowed to grow it becomes lobulated, causing unilateral enlargement and deformity of the face.

In the radiograph the chondroma is seen as a circumscribed semi-translucent area, spotted with calcified islands replacing the normal bone trabeculation. The tumour appears to be slowly overflowing its site of origin.

    4. *Central Fibroma* (ossifying fibroma).—This is not a common tumour and is rarely recognized in its original and basic form. In its growth it tends to change its internal formation to an ossifying fibroma or to a fibro-osteoma, and as such is more readily recognized.

The tumour is located more commonly in the mandible, is completely encapsulated, and easily shelled out.

Malignant Osteogenic Tumours.—These neoplasms are destructive and invasive. In their infiltration they present on the radiograph irregular osteolytic areas in that part of the bone which is involved.

    1. *Chondrosarcoma*.—The radiological differentiation between a benign chondroma and a chondrosarcoma may not be clearly shown. In the latter, all signs of encapsulation and limitation disappear, and irregular destruction of the bone becomes more apparent. The extension of the infiltrating mass into the immediate surrounding structure is an important diagnostic feature.

    2. *Myxoma*.—This is a soft central tumour, formed from undifferentiated retained embryonic osteogenic cells, which has become a mass of gelatinous substance.

It is found during the second and third decades of life, in both jaws, away from the tooth-bearing part of the mandible and maxilla. The tumour expands and destroys the bone, producing enlargement of the face, and often invades the oral cavity.

It presents a characteristic trabeculation formation often described as "honeycomb", is diffuse in its extent, and shows destruction of the cortex of the bone.

3. *Osteogenic Sarcoma.*—This is a rare entity. It is a solitary tumour occurring in either jaw, at any period of life, but mainly in the adolescent. There are many histological varieties.

Two types may be identified radiographically:—

a. *Osteolytic sarcoma*: Seen as irregular areas of bone destruction. In the shadow of the tumour there may be a limited amount of newly formed bone.

b. *Osteoblastic sarcoma*: The invasive and destructive activity of the tumour is accompanied by a high degree of bone production. It shows characteristic periosteal formation, with a palisade of bone spicules arranged at right angles to the bone cortex and producing a sun-ray effect.

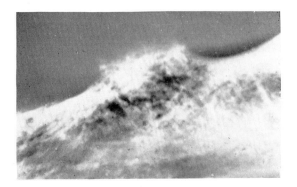

Fig. 663.—Exostosis. Bony out-growth from the alveolar margin in the edentulous $\overline{|45}$ region. Long history of an ill-fitting denture. The internal structure is of normal cancellous formation and continuous with that of the mandible.

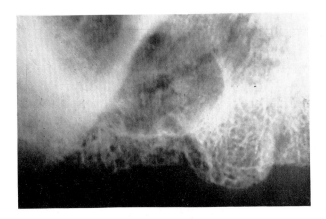

Fig. 664.—Exostosis. Local-ized peripheral circumscribed overgrowth of bone in the edentulous $\underline{|67}$ region. The cancellous composition of the lesion and its continuity with the maxillary bone are im-portant features.

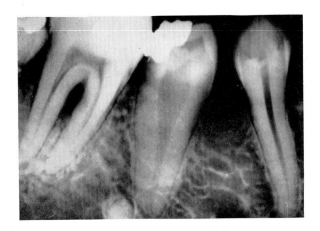

Fig. 665.—Enostosis. Local-ized small area of dense, non-cancellous bone, distal to the apex of $\overline{5|}$. This is a common site for such formations. No connexion with the apex of the $\overline{5|}$.

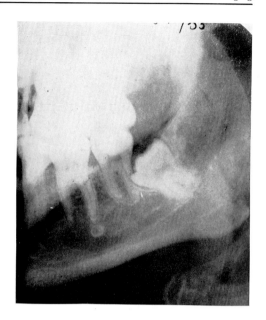

Fig. 666.—Enostosis. Unconnected with the apex of |6̄. May be mistaken for a cementoma.

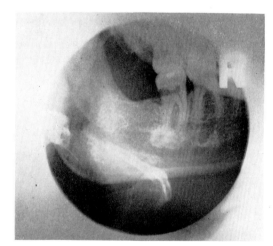

Fig. 667.—Enostosis. Irregular mass of dense, non-cancellous bone at apices of 7̄|. Not easily differentiated from sclerotic formation and ankylosis of the roots.

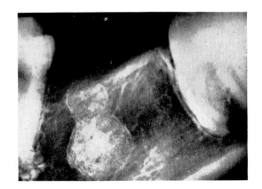

Fig. 668.—Enostosis. It is akin to an endosteal osteoma, having a well-defined capsule.

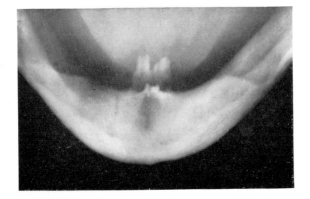

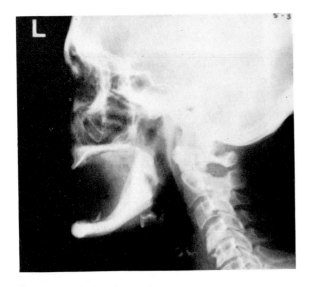

Fig. 669.—Exostosis of the genial tubercles. The occlusal view shows abnormally opaque, elongated, and enlarged genial tubercles. Seen more often in edentulous mandibles.

Fig. 670.—Exostosis of the genial tubercles. The lateral view depicts the genial tubercles detached and pulled backwards and upwards from behind the symphysis menti in an edentulous mandible.

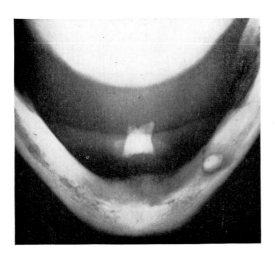

Fig. 671.—Exostosis of the genial tubercles. Occlusal view of *Fig.* 670. The detached tubercles are fused, highly opaque, and enlarged.

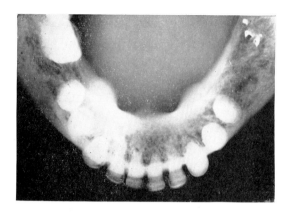

Fig. 672.—Torus mandibularis. Bilateral, dense, compact outgrowths of bone deposited on the inner surface of the mandible in the pre-molar regions, opposite the mental foramina.

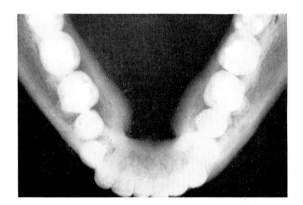

Fig. 673.—Torus mandibularis. The bilateral opaque tori extend along the inner wall of the mandible from the canine to the second molar regions. They are forming two bony shelves converging over the floor of the mouth.

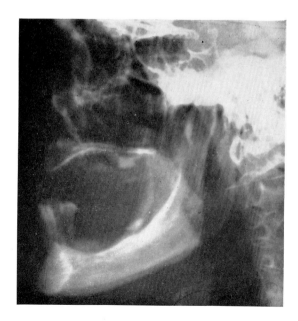

Fig. 674.—Torus palatinus. The lateral view reveals the localized, opaque, bony protuberance attached to the posterior part of the hard palate. It is growing into the oral cavity, suspended from the roof of the mouth.

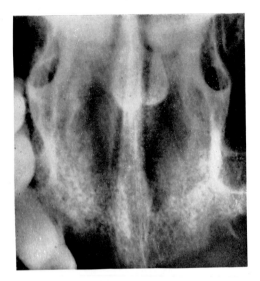

Fig. 675.—Torus palatinus. The occlusal view shows the double lobulated growth in the midline of the posterior part of the hard palate.

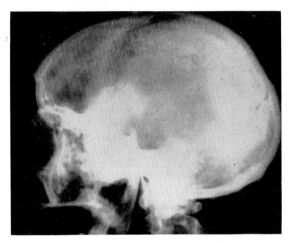

Fig. 676.—Hyperostosis cranii. Irregular proliferation of the inner table of the bones of the vault. The condition is symptomless and may be due to disturbance of the endocrine system. Often seen at the menopause or in old people.

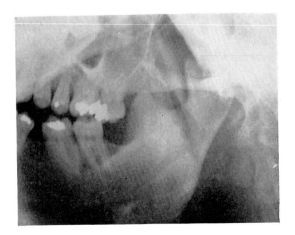

Fig. 677.—Hyperostosis of the condyle. Enlargement of the condylar head, broadening of the neck of the condyle, narrowing of the mandibular notch, and the coronoid process slightly under-developed.

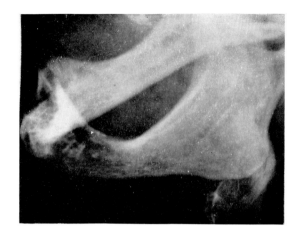

Fig. 678.—Hyperostosis of the mandibular angle. Enlargement of the angle of the jaw and the lower half of the ascending ramus.

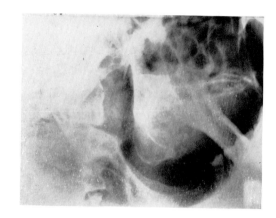

Fig. 679.—Hyperostosis of the maxillary tuberosity. Diffuse overgrowth of the upper jaw involving the molar region and tuberosity. The cortex is expanding and the bone is growing downwards and backwards.

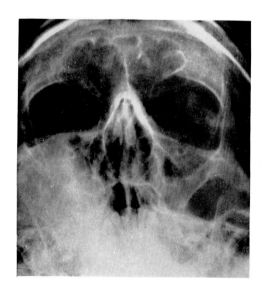

Fig. 680.—Hyperostosis of the right maxilla. Uniform opacity of the body of the right maxilla and of the malar bone. The right antral cavity is partially obliterated, and the floor of the right orbit is curved upwards.

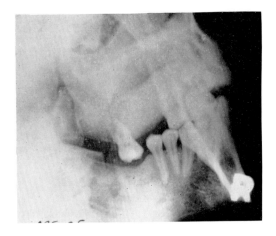

Fig. 681.—The lateral oblique view of *Fig.* 680 demonstrates the massive involvement of the right maxilla.

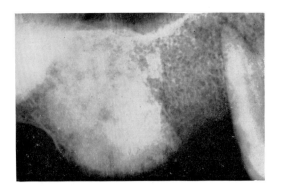

Fig. 682.—Osteoma. There is a central osteoma in the 765| region. The radio-opacity is not completely homogeneous, and is probably of the fibro-osteoma type. The tumour appears to be encapsulated.

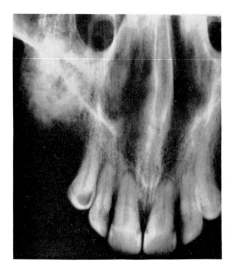

Fig. 683.—Occlusal view of *Fig.* 682. This confirms the impression that the lesion is circumscribed and encapsulated, and the variation of the internal density is well shown.

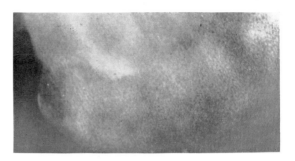

Fig. 684.—Osteoma. There is marked enlargement of the molar region and tuberosity of the right maxilla. The internal uniform compact formation shows no demarcation from the surrounding main bone.

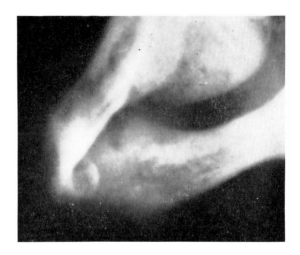

Fig. 685.—Osteoma durum. This large ivory-like formation involves the premolar and molar regions of the left maxilla.

Fig. 686.—Osteoma. The bony new growth appears to be confined to the alveolar region incorporating 76543|. The floor of the antrum can still be seen.

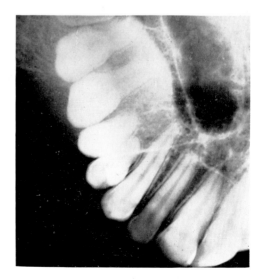

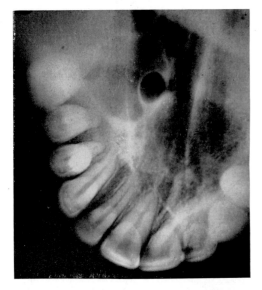

Fig. 687.—Osteoma. The tumour is benign in character and in its growth is seen displacing the nasolacrimal opening.

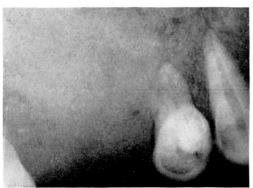

Fig. 688.—Osteoma. The radiograph presents a shadow of fine stippling, often described as resembling the texture of orange peel.

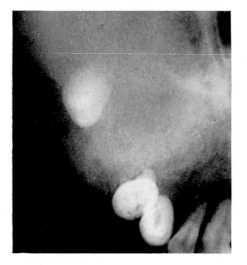

Fig. 689.—Osteoma. Occlusal view of *Fig.* 688 showing complete envelopment of the 8|.

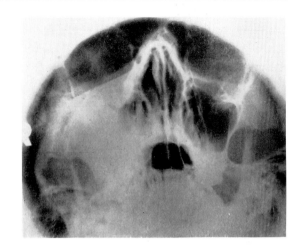

Fig. 690.—Osteoma. Almost total obliteration of the right maxillary sinus. The outer wall of the antrum is sharp and clearly delineated with no expansion or distension.

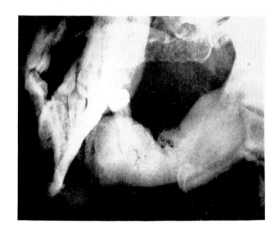

Fig. 691.—Osteoma durum. Radio-opaque mass in $\overline{|345678}$ region of solid, compact bone. It has a fairly sharp margin mesially, and is limited by the inferior dental canal which is displaced towards the inferior border of the mandible.

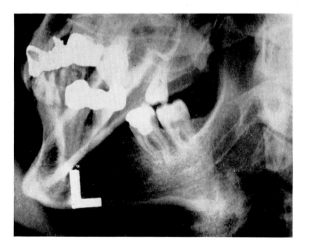

Fig. 692.—Extra-osseous osteoma. A cancellated mass with a broad base is protruding from the angle of the left mandible. The patient was a professional boxer and the lesion is probably a traumatic osteoma.

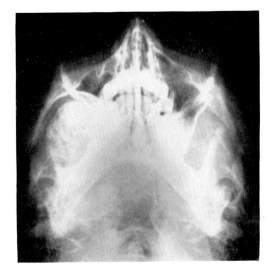

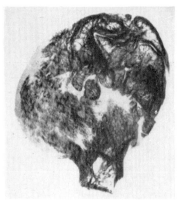

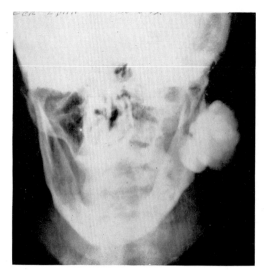

Fig. 693.—Condylar osteoma. Large pedunculated bony mass attached to the base of the neck of the mandibular condyle on the right side.

Fig. 694.—Radiograph of the pedunculated osteoma shown in *Fig.* 693 after excision. This type is sometimes described as an osteochondroma or even an exostosis.

Fig. 695.—Pedunculated osteoma. The postero-anterior view shows a large lobulated osteoma attached by a "stalk" to the outer surface of the ramus just below the base of the condylar process.

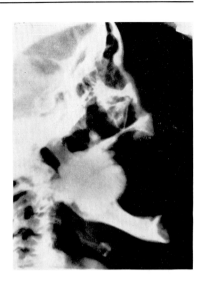

Fig. 696.—Lateral view of *Fig.* 695. This view emphasizes the massive structure of the osteoma. It gives, however, the impression that the growth is incorporated in the general osseous formation of the ramus.

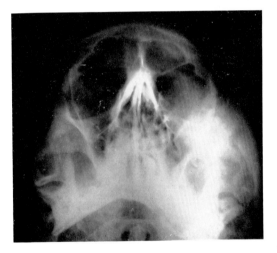

Figs. 697, 698.—Osteoma durum and osteoma spongiosum. This patient was torpedoed when serving in the Merchant Navy and was rendered unconscious when hit by a floating spar while swimming away from the ship. Within twelve months he developed an osteoma of his left malar bone and the postero-external surface of the left maxilla. The circumscribed lesion in the $\overline{|4567}$ region is an osteoma spongiosum.

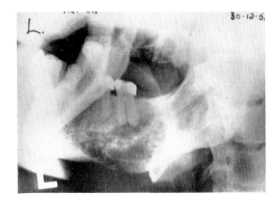

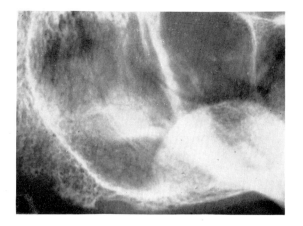

Fig. 699.—Osteoma in the maxillary antrum. Dome-shaped, sessile opacity on the floor of the maxillary sinus. The benign osteoma exhibits a cancellous bone structure.

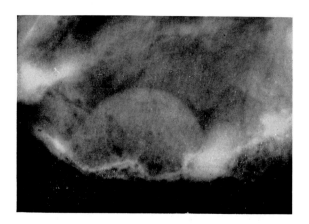

Fig. 700.—Osteoma in the maxillary antrum. Posterior to the basal osteoma is the retained root of |8. The cloudiness of the antral shadow is indicative of an associated secondary infection of the maxillary sinus.

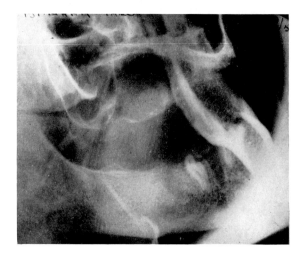

Fig. 701.—Oblique lateral view of *Fig.* 700.

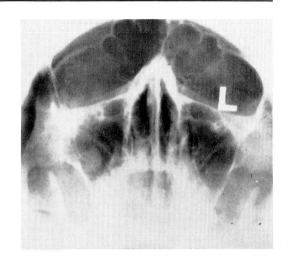

Fig. 702.—Osteoma in the maxillary antrum. A pedunculated osteoma is seen attached to the inner side of the outer wall of the right antrum.

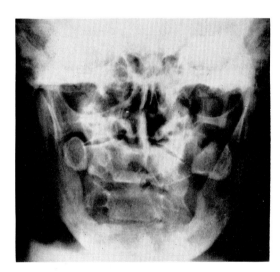

Figs. 703, 704.—Multiple osteomata. There are a number of osteomata in the upper jaw of this edentulous patient.

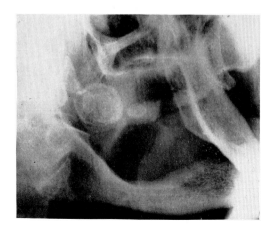

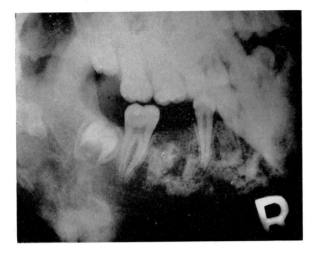

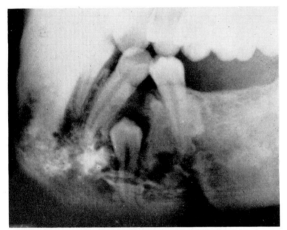

Figs. 705, 706.—Multiple osteomata in a girl, aged 12 years. Scattered, ill-defined areas of different sizes of radio-opacity in the mandible. There were no lesions in the maxilla. The patient's grandmother was similarly affected.

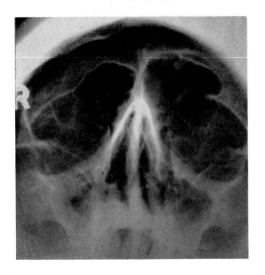

Fig. 707.—Osteoma of the frontal sinus. Pedunculated osteoma arising from the roof of the left orbit. Osteomata in the frontal sinus are fairly common lesions.

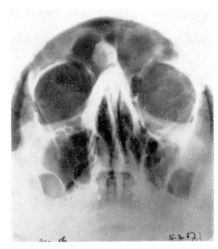

Fig. 708.—Osteoma of the frontal sinus. Large ivory osteoma in the right frontal sinus at the midline.

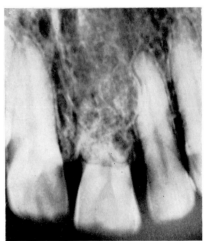

Fig. 709.—Chondroma. The entire root of |1 has been resorbed, together with its supporting bone. The root and alveolar bone have been replaced by a circumscribed, semitranslucent area, containing multiple calcified areas. The lesion shows a well-defined outline and is encapsulated.

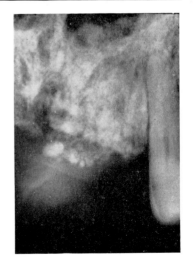

Fig. 710.—Chondrosarcoma. Female patient, aged 54 years. |12 region depicts a mottled area of indefinite calcification and rarefaction, with many isolated discrete marginal bodies. An important feature is the extension of the new growth into the floor of the left nasal fossa.

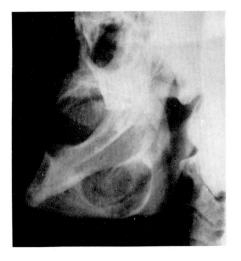

Fig. 711.—Central fibroma (ossifying fibroma). The lateral oblique view presents a large radiolucent, non-trabeculated area in the $\overline{|5678}$ region, with a well-defined margin. There are a number of small opaque bodies within the tumour shadow indicative of active ossification.

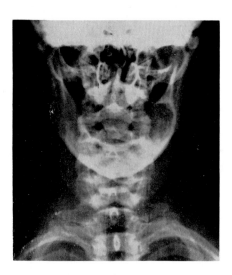

Fig. 712.—The postero-anterior view of *Fig.* 711 shows some thinning of the cortex of the body of the mandible with a mild degree of expansion.

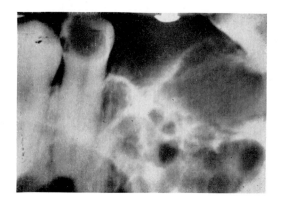

Fig. 713.—Osteogenic myxoma. $\overline{|4567}$ region shows an expanding, pseudo-multiloculated appearance of the honeycomb type. Microscopic examination resulted in a diagnosis of fibromyxoma.

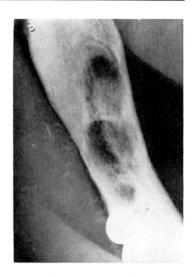

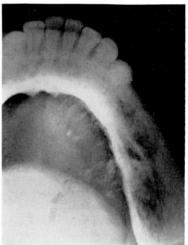

Fig. 714, 715.—Osteogenic sarcoma. The occlusal view reveals destructive rarefaction of the mandible in the premolar region involving both walls. An important feature is the sun-ray effect of periosteal formation against the periphery of the bone, lingually and buccally.

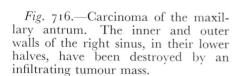

Fig. 716.—Carcinoma of the maxillary antrum. The inner and outer walls of the right sinus, in their lower halves, have been destroyed by an infiltrating tumour mass.

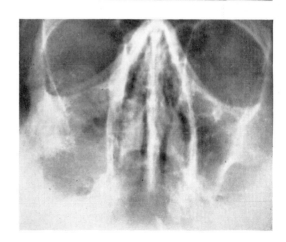

Intra-osseous or Central Tumours

THESE tumours are formed from tissues within the jaws and arise from: (1) Cells in the medulla. (2) Blood-vessels and lymphatics. (3) Nerve tissues. (4) Metastatic deposition.

1. Central Giant-cell Tumour.—This is a solitary cellular lesion, benign in character, arising from cells contained in the bone-marrow. It differs from the giant-cell epulis, which is peripheral in its position and occurs on the gingiva.

Similar, but multiple, lesions are found in generalized osteitis fibrosa due to hyperparathyroidism.

The giant-cell tumour which occurs in children during the period of dentition is known as an odontoclastoma, is found along the alveolus, and when encapsulated simulates a dental cyst.

The true central giant-cell tumour is not encapsulated and infiltrates the surrounding structures. It is frequently seen between the ages of 15 and 25 years, and is found in the canine region of the maxilla, at the symphysis menti, and in the mandibular premolar area.

The tumour produces expansion of the bone and may cause marked unilateral deformity of the face. The teeth may become separated and loose.

The radiograph of a central giant-cell tumour is variable, but in the main, depicts the lesion as an area of multiple osteolytic foci and of a cystic appearance. The margins are irregular in outline, showing infiltrating activity, and the lesion tends to displace the teeth, which may exhibit apical resorption.

2. An Angioma of the Jaw is a vascular neoplasm found in the bone, and is distinct from the hæmangioma located in the soft tissue of the mouth.

The central type of angioma forms from blood-vessels in the medullary spaces and is a rare lesion.

The peripheral type arises from the vessels of the attached periosteum, invades and destroys the outer surfaces of the bone, and gradually involves the cancellous region.

Both types of angioma occur at any age, are benign in character, and of slow growth. They may produce a limited amount of bone expansion.

3. Ewing's Tumour.—This is an endothelial myeloma and it arises from the endothelial lining of blood-vessels and lymphatics. There are many different histological types and they are found more often in the long bones than in the jaws.

This is not a common neoplasm and it tends to metastasize.

The lesion occurs in children and young adults, at the symphysis menti, the horizontal body of the mandible, and at the angle of the jaw. In the maxilla it is the antrum which is the site of predilection.

The radiograph simulates chronic osteomyelitis with diffuse involvement of the bone. The cortex of the bone is often split into layers and shows expansion.

The tumour mass may contain osteophytic outgrowths extending from the main bone.

4. Multiple Myeloma.—The lesion found in the jaw is only one manifestation of a multiplicity of similar tumours scattered throughout the various bones of the skeleton, in the same patient. It is formed from myelocytes, lymphocytes, and red blood-cells located in the bone-marrow. The maxilla is rarely involved.

The age incidence is between 40 and 70 years, and in many cases the lesion is found during routine X-ray examination or after a spontaneous fracture. Radiography is of the utmost value in these cases, especially that of the skull.

In the mandible the most common situation is the angle of the jaw, where multiple, small, rounded, radiolucent areas are seen around and below the inferior dental canal. As the disease progresses the hollow areas grow bigger, fuse with each other, and form larger rarefied lesions.

The long bones, ribs, and skull show punched-out, rounded, radiolucent areas of varying diameters, and there is no increase in the thickness of the bone. On the other hand, the cortex suffers neither destruction nor expansion.

5. Neurogenic Tumours are formed from nerve tissue and perineural tissue within the bone. They include neuromas, neurogenic fibromas, and fibrosarcomas, and it must be left to the histopathologist to determine their exact nature.

These tumours are not common, and they are solitary entities with a predilection for the mandibular premolar region.

The benign type appears on the radiograph as a radiolucent area in the premolar–molar region, very well defined, and lying on the buccal aspect. It simulates a periodontal cyst.

The malignant type loses its sharp margin, and the osteolytic character is seen as the rarefied area extends into the surrounding tissue and eventually produces expansion of the bone.

6. Metastatic Tumours in the jaws are relatively rare. The secondary lesions reaching the jaws via the blood-stream grow diffusely in the medulla, and their osteolytic activity results in gross bone changes.

The radiographic picture varies from irregular areas of rarefaction to pseudocystic formations. The osteolytic areas usually suggest osteomyelitis; in other cases, there is bone expansion and occasionally even bone deposition.

The cortex of the bone may become perforated and result in a pathological fracture.

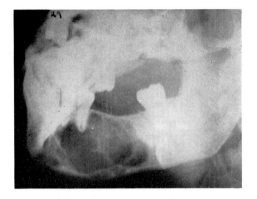

Fig. 717.—Benign central giant-cell tumour in a female, aged 25 years. Well-outlined, lobulated, and trabeculated radiolucent area in $\overline{|4567}$ region. Mild resorption of the apices $\overline{|45}$.

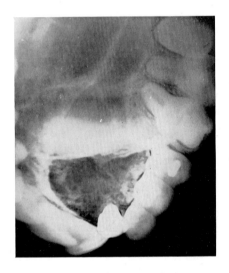

Fig. 718.—Benign central giant-cell tumour in a male, aged 17 years, $\underline{|123}$ region. This lobulated radiolucent area is suggestive of a globulomaxillary cyst, and was later identified by the histopathologist.

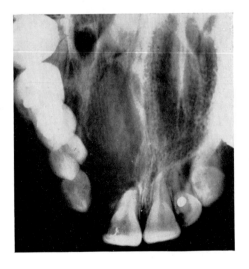

Fig. 719.—Benign central giant-cell tumour, $\underline{321|}$ region. The tumour has grown and extended half-way along the long axis of the hard palate and shows some expansion laterally.

Fig. 720.—Odontoclastoma in a boy, aged 8 years. Lower left incisor region. $\overline{123|}$ are unerupted, and the retained $\overline{bc|}$ show a crescentic resorption of their roots. The radiolucent area between $\overline{b|}$ and the unerupted $\overline{2|}$ is cystic, and fan-like spiculated bone is growing into it.

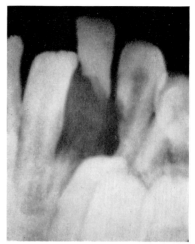

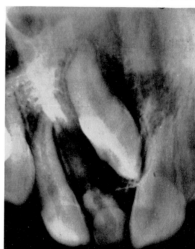

Fig. 721.—Odontoclastoma in a girl, aged 11 years. $1|$ region.

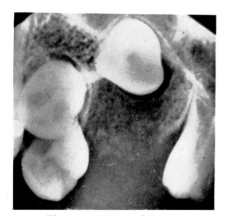

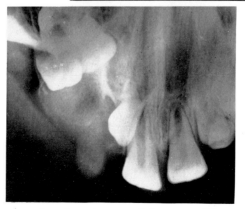

Figs. 722, 723.—Odontoclastoma, $32|$ region, in a boy aged 8 years. All deciduous teeth in this area were shed two years earlier. $3|$ unerupted, $4|$ displaced laterally. No encapsulation, but bone expansion well seen.

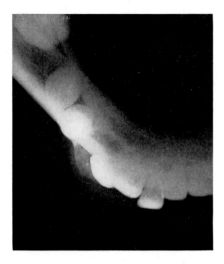

Fig. 724.—Odontoclastoma in a girl, aged 15 years. $\overline{43|}$ region. Occlusal view reveals the swelling in the $\overline{43|}$ region. Many of the other bones of the skeleton were radiographed, but showed no changes. This was a solitary lesion.

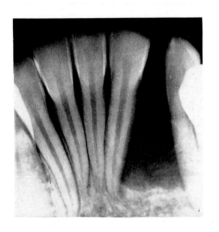

Fig. 725.—Odontoclastoma in a girl, aged 12 years. Coronal divarication of the lower left lateral incisor and canine teeth, with total loss of the interdental bony structure. No sign of any new bone formation within the soft-tissue mass which is lying in the deep scooped-out hollow excavation between the teeth.

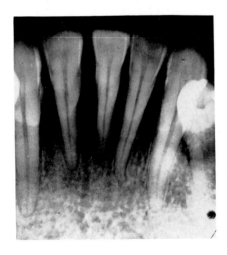

Fig. 726.—Peripheral osteoclastoma in a female, aged 45 years. No pathognomonic signs in the radiograph of a tumour. Recession and resorption of the alveolar bone margin with no separation of the teeth.

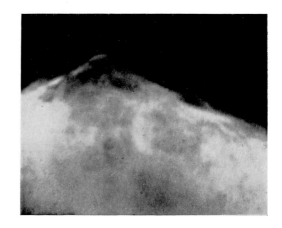

Fig. 727.—Angioma in $\overline{21|12}$ region. The lesion is centrally placed in the bone. There is an indication of expansion of the bone at its free alveolar margin.

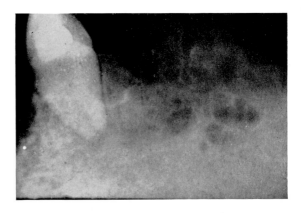

Fig. 728.—Peripheral angioma in $\overline{|456}$ region. "Soap-bubble" appearance produced in the alveolar bone.

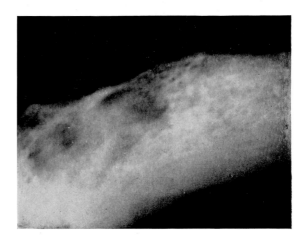

Fig. 729.—Angioma in $\overline{|123}$ region. The cortex of the mandible has been destroyed and the lesion is involving the cancellous bone.

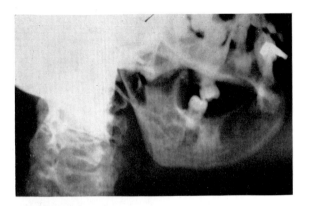

Fig. 730.—Myelomatosis. The body and ascending ramus of the left mandible presents multiple small radiolucent areas around and below the inferior dental canal. There are many radiolucent areas in the bodies of the cervical vertebræ.

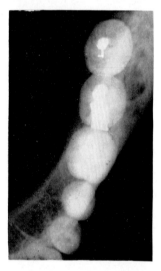

Figs. 731–739.—Myelomatosis in the same patient.

Fig. 731.—Occlusal view shows numerous small radiolucent areas lying on the buccal side of the molar region of the left mandible.

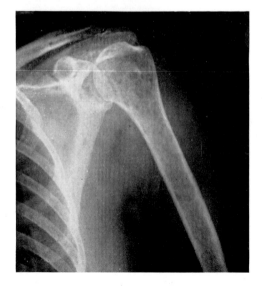

Fig. 732.—The multiple, small, rounded, radiolucent areas in the humerus simulate mottling of the bone. The outer cortical bone shows no change.

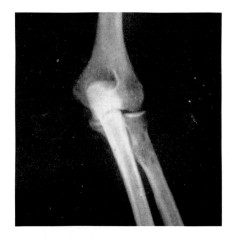

Fig. 733.—The upper end of the left radius is punctuated by many small discrete rounded areas due to local myelomatous osteolysis.

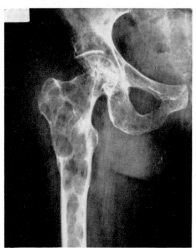

Fig. 734.—The right innominate bone and the upper end of the right femur are involved by the disease. The lesions in the upper part of the femur are fusing to form larger radiolucent areas over a greater extent of the bone. The bone is beginning to expand as the cortex becomes thinner.

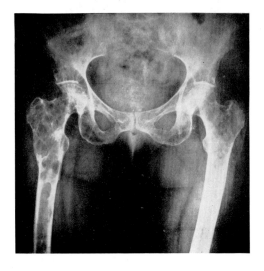

Fig. 735.—All the bones of the pelvis show extensive distribution of the disease. The upper end of the left femur is also involved.

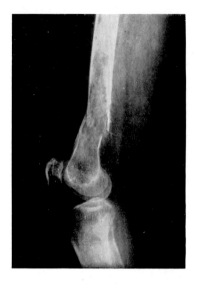

Fig. 736.—The lower part of the right femur is almost devoid of medullary trabeculation and the weakened bone presents a pathological fracture.

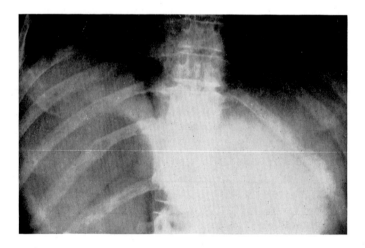

Fig. 737.—All the lower ribs are riddled with myelomatous lesions.

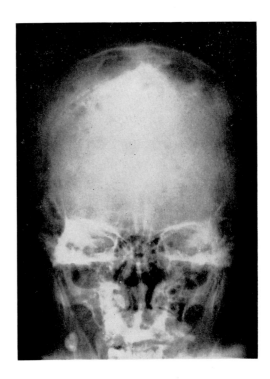

Figs. 738, 739.—Lateral and postero-anterior views of the skull. Multiple punched-out areas in the calvarium. No increase in the width of the tables of the skull. Complete absence of any osteoblastic activity.

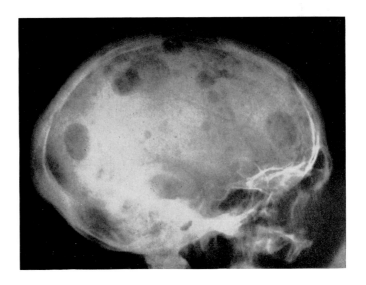

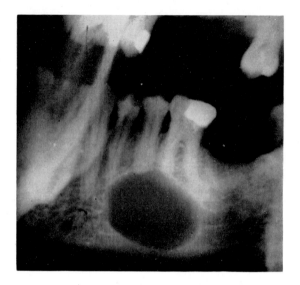

Fig. 740.—Neurofibroma. Radio-lucent area below the apices of $\overline{|56}$ simulating a periodontal cyst. The main indication of its nature is the fact that the inferior dental canal abruptly terminates at the margin of the lesion and does not run through the radiolucent area.

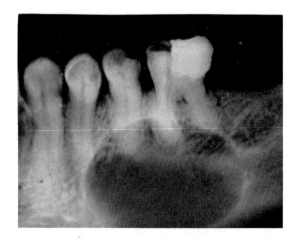

Fig. 741.—Neurofibroma. Well-defined radiolucent area in $\overline{|56}$ region. The outer wall is not continuous with the laminæ dura of the teeth.

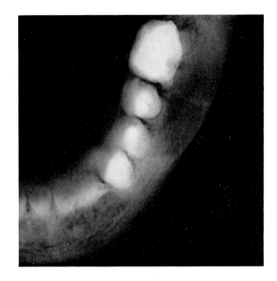

Fig. 742.—Neurofibroma. Occlusal view of *Fig.* 741 which shows that the radio-lucent area lies on the buccal aspect of the teeth.

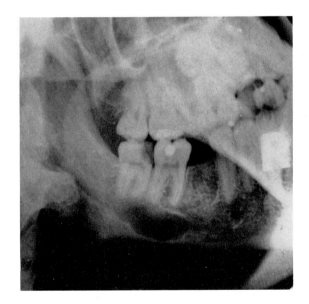

Fig. 743.—Neurofibroma. The irregular radiolucent area below the $\overline{87|}$ is an enlargement of the proximal end of the inferior dental canal. The continuation of the canal is seen extending to the mental foramen.

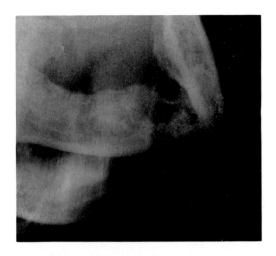

Fig. 744.—Metastatic deposit from primary carcinoma of the thyroid gland. Irregular area of bone destruction in $\overline{543|}$ region. Although the margin of the area is ill-defined, the general outline is circular.

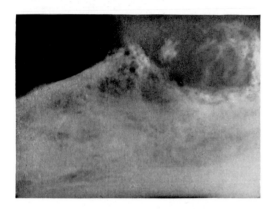

Fig. 745.—Metastatic deposit. Primary focus in the prostate. Irregular area of rarefaction in $\overline{|67}$ region with pseudocystic formation.

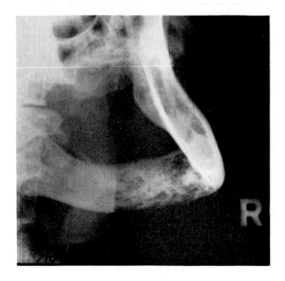

Fig. 746.—Metastatic deposit. Primary focus in the prostate. Osteolytic involvement of the body of the right mandible, simulating osteomyelitis. Erosion of the lower border of the mandible.

Soft-tissue Tumours of the Oral Cavity

ALL histological varieties of soft-tissue tumours of the oral cavity form from the oral mucosa and other soft tissue in and around the cavity. The majority are peripheral outgrowths, pedunculated or sessile, found in either sulcus. Some creep in between the teeth and displace the crowns; others invade and infiltrate the immediate structures, involving the gingivæ and later the alveolar process and even the main bone.

Soft-tissue neoplasms do not cast a shadow on a radiograph unless an X-ray beam of low penetration is employed. Even so, there is but little value in undertaking any radiographic examination in these cases. On the other hand, when the tumours lie against the teeth and produce divarication of the crowns, a radiograph may be helpful.

It is not proposed to enumerate the many varieties of soft-tissue tumours, nor yet to describe them. It should suffice to discuss those entities which produce secondary effects on the more opaque structures in and around the mouth, and which present recognizable radiographic changes.

1. Hyperplasia is not a true neoplasm, but is one of the most common swellings seen in the mouth. It is an overgrowth of the gums and is composed of organized chronic inflammatory granulation tissue. The lesion may be widespread along the upper and lower jaws or be confined to a limited area on the alveolar margin. No radiographic changes can be seen until the marginal periodontal membrane becomes involved, and then the radiograph will reveal the extent of erosion, destruction, and resorption of the underlying osseous structure. The teeth may be loosened when deprived of their supporting bone, and although they will probably alter in inclination they will not be displaced.

Calcification or ossification does not take place within the inflamed overgrowth of soft tissue.

2. Fibroid Epulis.—The true growths, benign and malignant, arise from any of the constituent tissue formations found in the mouth, and are classified as epulides. In reality, these lesions are peripheral fibromas. They arise from the deep layers of the mucosa, the periodontal membrane, or from the periosteum of the mandible or maxilla. There seems to be sufficient justification to call them "fibroid epulides".

Ossification and calcification may be observed in these new growths, when they are termed "ossifying fibromas".

3. Osteoclastoma (peripheral giant-cell tumour).—This neoplasm originates in the alveolar dental periosteum which is osteoblastic tissue. The tumour grows as a result of excess activity of normal bone-forming function. It is a solitary tumour, benign in character, and in no way associated with such similar growths as are seen in osteitis fibrosa.

Many of these tumours occur in children during the period of dentition and are called "odontoclastoma". They present X-ray appearances sufficiently definite to differentiate them from those neoplasms seen in the older patient (p. 324).

4. Fibrosarcoma is a rare, but highly malignant tumour which arises from the alveolar periosteum or periodontal membrane. The malignant infiltration into the bone is often rapid and uneven, so that the radiograph reveals an irregular, serrated bone margin penetrating deep into the main bone, leaving a trail of many isolated small bone sequestra in the wake of the invading growth.

The image of the tumour shows no spur formation, no spiculation, and no deposits of chondrification or ossification. Standing teeth became loose and gradually separate from their normal vertical alinement and are displaced laterally with a parallel separation.

5. Hæmangioma is formed from the endothelium of blood-vessels. It is a common tumour occurring in the oral cavity and may be multiple. Although the hæmangioma is benign it may invade the underlying bone and cause osteolysis. Phleboliths may form in the swelling and show in the radiograph as concentric calcification deposits in line formation along the veins which contain thrombi.

6. Mucoceles and Epidermoid Tumours.—These entities are found on the inner surface of the lips and cheek, on the soft palate, and in the buccal mucosa of both sulci. As they are interposed between the X-ray beam and intra-oral film, their shadows are superimposed on the radiograph and may be mistaken for dental cysts and other lesions. A mucocele is a retention cyst formed by the occlusion of the outlet of the excretory duct of a mucous gland and is usually of traumatic origin. A ranula is a retention cyst of the submaxillary duct. A muco-epidermoid tumour arises from the cells of the mucous ducts.

7. Carcinoma may occur anywhere in the oral cavity arising from the epithelial lining cells. It may invade the bones of the maxilla and mandible from primary sites on the gingival mucosa. Carcinoma of the alveolar gingiva is frequently located in the mandibular third molar region, and in its growth causes extensive destruction of the posterior portion of the mandible and of the anterior part of the ascending ramus. A primary carcinoma may begin in the submandibular gland and extend upwards to the lower border of the mandible, producing widespread infiltration and eventual pathological fracture.

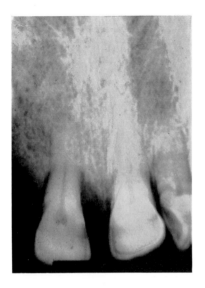

Fig. 747.—Hyperplasia of the gingiva. Irregular erosion and destruction of the alveolar margin around the proximal part of 1| socket. Resorption of the bony interdental septum between the upper central incisors.

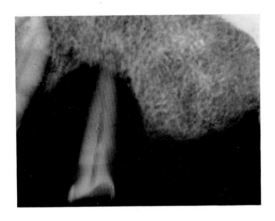

Fig. 748.—Hyperplasia of the gingiva. The |2 is surrounded and almost submerged by a localized massive overgrowth of the gum tissue, which is of an inflammatory character.

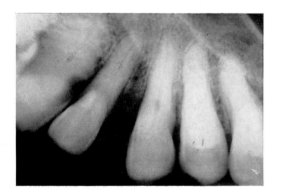

Fig. 749.—Fibroid epulis. Separation of the crowns of |2 and |3 with widening of the proximal part of the bony interdental septum. The rarefaction of the interproximal bone is due to pressure atrophy of the neoplasm.

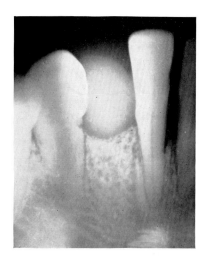

Fig. 750.—Fibroid epulis. A globular mass of soft tissue is seen on the free concave margin of the alveolar bone between $\overline{2|}$ and $\overline{4|}$. The $\overline{3|}$ is absent. A beam of low penetration was employed.

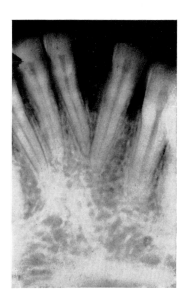

Fig. 751.—Fibroid epulis. Widening and flattening of the summit of the bony interdental septum between the $\overline{|1}$ and $\overline{|2}$. Marked pivotal divarication of the crowns of the teeth.

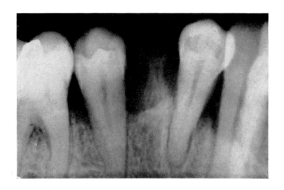

Fig. 752.—Fibroid epulis. $\overline{54|}$ region. Bony spur from free alveolar margin extending into soft mass of epulis, with tooth divarication.

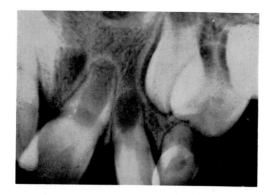

Fig. 753.—Fibroid epulis in a girl, aged 8 years. Small interdental bony spur with pivotal divarication. The upper left incisor teeth are impacted against their immediate neighbouring teeth.

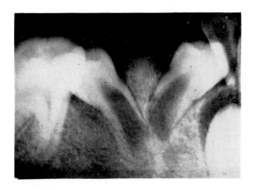

Fig. 754.—Fibroid epulis in a girl, aged 10 years. Divarication of the lower right un-erupted premolar teeth with impaction against neighbouring teeth.

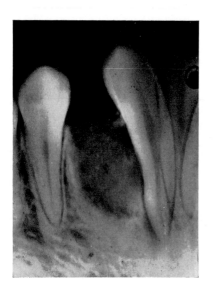

Fig. 755.—Ossifying fibroma. Numerous small irregular-shaped opacities within the translucent area of the epulis. Marked displacement of the canine tooth from the first lower right premolar tooth.

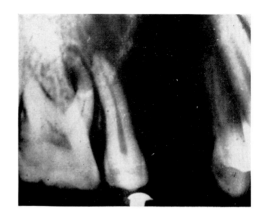

Fig. 756.—Peripheral fibrosarcoma in a male, aged 19 years. Marked destruction of the alveolar bone leaving the teeth "floating in the breeze". Parallel separation of the premolar teeth.

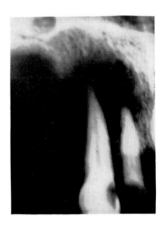

Fig. 757.—Peripheral fibrosarcoma in a male, aged 55 years. The teeth appear unsupported, but still retain their vertical disposition. The irregular destruction of the alveolar bone is most marked.

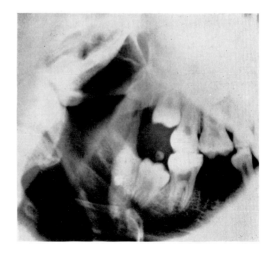

Fig. 758.—Hæmangioma of the cheek. Laminated calcified bodies of a whorled appearance as superimposed shadows seen in the molar region above the image of the unerupted $\overline{8|}$ and overlying the inferior dental canal.

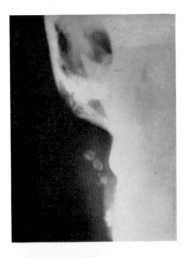

Fig. 759.—Hæmangioma of the cheek. Postero-anterior view of *Fig.* 758 showing the chain of small rounded opacities lying external to the ascending ramus of the mandible.

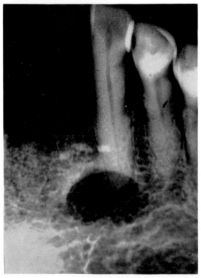

Fig. 760.—Mucocele. Superimposed shadow of a retention cyst located on the inner surface of the lower lip in the left canine region. No outer wall image. The bone structure is clearly seen through the cyst.

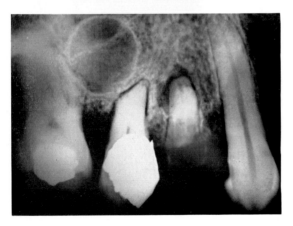

Fig. 761.—Mucocele. The alveolar bone trabeculation and the shadow of the lower part of the maxillary antrum are discernible through the cyst.

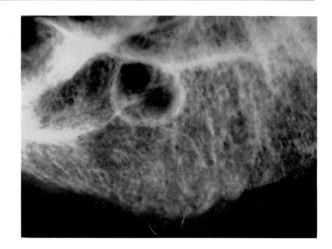

Fig. 762.—Muco-epidermoid tumour. This was a semi-solid lesion firmly attached to the alveolar process below the outer wall of the floor of the maxillary sinus. Note the thickened cortical wall of the tumour.

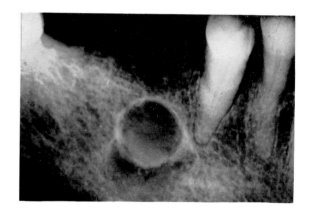

Fig. 763.—Muco-epidermoid tumour. This entity was deep-seated in a hollow of the outer wall of the mandible. It was adherent to the bone. There are signs of some osteolytic activity around and below the tumour.

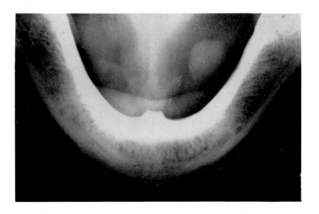

Fig. 764.—Ranula. A retention cyst of the proximal end of the left submaxillary duct.

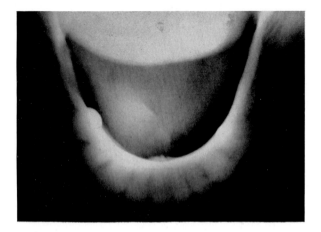

Fig. 765.—Sublingual retention cyst.

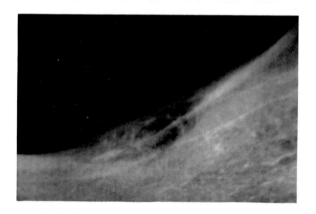

Fig. 766.—Carcinoma in a female, aged 64 years. A soft-tissue mass is seen in the $\overline{|67}$ region with an underlying elliptical area of rarefaction of the bone along its free margin.

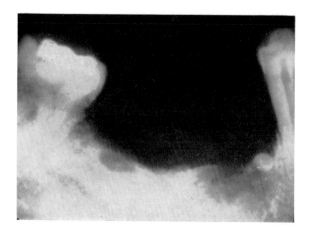

Fig. 767.—Carcinoma in a male, aged 75 years. $\overline{76|}$ region shows a soft-tissue shadow above the alveolar margin which reveals erosion of its free edge. There is an infiltrating rarefaction of the bone beyond.

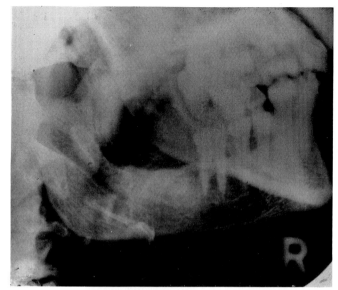

Fig. 768.—Carcinoma in a female, aged 51 years. Erosion and destruction of the anterior border of the right ascending ramus.

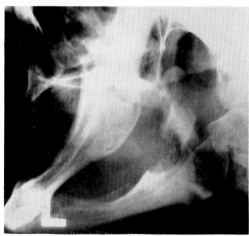

Fig. 769.—Carcinoma in a male, aged 79 years. Digital erosion in $\overline{8}$ region with active osteolysis.

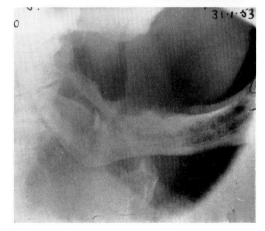

Fig. 770.—Carcinoma in a male, aged 80 years. Massive and extensive destruction of the mandible from the lower right third molar region, along the ascending ramus anterior to the inferior dental canal and the coronoid process.

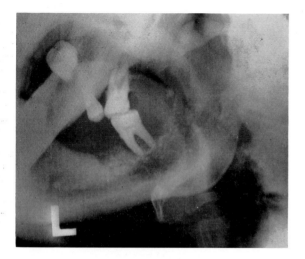

Fig. 771.—Carcinoma in a male, aged 68 years. The mandible, from the lower left second molar region up the ramus to the mandibular notch, presents a deep area of rarefaction, as if washed clear by an advancing tide.

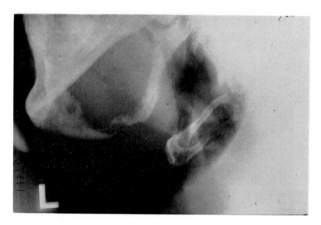

Fig. 772.—Carcinoma in a male, aged 71 years. Almost complete destruction of the mandible from the lower left premolar region to the mandibular notch. Pathological fracture.

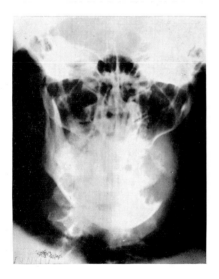

Fig. 773.—Postero-anterior view of *Fig.* 772. This demonstrates the massive involvement of the mandible with no displacement of the fragments coincident with the pathological fracture. The fragments are kept in position by the enveloping large neoplastic mass.

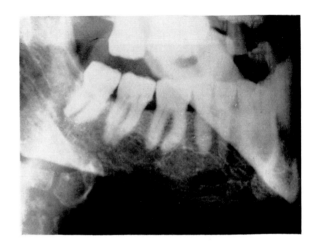

Fig. 774.—Carcinoma of the sub-mandibular gland in a male, aged 72 years. There is a triangular invasion and destruction of the lower border of the mandible in the $\overline{76|}$ region.

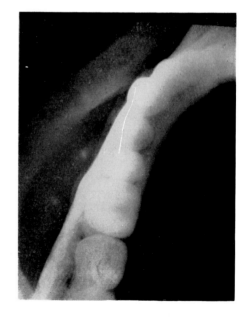

Fig. 775.—Occlusal view of Fig. 774. The upward growth of the malignant neoplasm of the sub-mandibular gland is stripping the platysma and soft tissue of the face off the bone whilst maintaining a close envelopment of the mandible.

Systemic Diseases

GENERALIZED systemic disease affects the jaws and teeth in a similar manner and produces changes closely allied to those seen in the other bones of the skeleton.

In most cases the growth of the bone may be enfeebled and even arrested; in others there may be acceleration of osteoblastic activity with new bone formation. Interference with calcium metabolism is a characteristic feature.

Many lesions have a congenital or hereditary aetiology, are found in early life, and affect the skeleton during the period of growth and development. Others are seen in later periods of adult life, and certain diseases appear to have a predilection for specific bones.

Routine and specialized radiographic techniques demonstrate the amount of interference in skeletal growth, the distribution of the lesions, the degree of decalcification, the presence of fracture, and the resultant healed deformities.

In a few diseases the facial changes are the more prominent features and readily recognized, and the radiograph becomes almost pathognomonic.

Systemic diseases may be considered under the following headings:—
1. Nutritional diseases.
2. Endocrine disturbances.
3. Osteodystrophies.

1. In Nutritional Diseases such as general ill-health, rickets, and infantile scurvy, radiography is of great value in determining the amount of retardation of skeletal growth of the child, and of uncalcified trabeculation. There may be delayed eruption of the permanent teeth and these may reveal hypoplastic defects. After eruption, the teeth may show abnormal spacing and malocclusion.

2. Endocrine Disturbances often produce spectacular changes in the jaws and teeth. In many cases no radiographic changes can be noted.

a. *Thyroid Gland.*—
i. In *hypothyroidism* there is a peculiar lateral development of the face, with retarded growth of the facial bones and delayed eruption of the teeth.
ii. In *hyperthyroidism* there are no specific bone changes, but the deciduous teeth may exfoliate early with accelerated eruption of the permanent dentition.

b. *Pituitary Gland.*—
i. In *hypopituitarism* or *infantilism*, the radiograph usually shows small facial bones and irregularities in dentition.
ii. In *hyperpituitarism* or *gigantism* the radiograph shows proportional enlargement of the bones of the skeleton, including the jaws and teeth.
iii. *Acromegaly* is a disease associated with a pituitary tumour and occurs between the ages of 20 and 40 years. A number of distinctive features are seen in the radiograph:—
The head is hexagonal in shape.
The sella turcica is enlarged with signs of destruction.

The mandible develops an obtuse angle and protrudes.
The condylar head is enlarged.
The teeth are spaced and often in version.

c. Parathyroid Gland.—

i. In *hypoparathyroidism* radiography is not markedly informative. Some degree of underdevelopment of the premaxilla is usually apparent with an open bite. Hypoplasia of the teeth is a common feature.

ii. In *hyperparathyroidism* (osteitis fibrosa cystica) there is a generalized decalcification of the skeleton. It is found commonly in the middle-aged, and the first recognizable lesion is in the jaws. The mandible and maxilla present a picture of extensive osteoporosis with multiple cystic areas, which are osteoclastomas. The cortex is thinned and there is gross expansion of the bone. Many bones, including the skull, are involved simultaneously in the same patient. The teeth are highly calcified and show little signs of caries. They tend to drift and produce abnormal spacing, and there is pronounced malocclusion.

3. Osteodystrophies (or fibrous dysplasia of bone).—A number of conditions involving the skeleton and in particular the facial bones, of unknown origin, are described under this classification.

a. Fibrocystic Disease (cherubism).—The medullary portion of the bone is replaced by fibrous tissue. There is diffuse involvement of one or more bones, and when the facial bones are affected bilaterally, in a child, the condition is described as cherubism.

It is a perverted activity of bone formation, starting in early life and of slow development. Members of the same family may be affected, but there is no generalized decalcification of the skeleton.

The jaws are often involved, and the radiograph shows a rarefied trabeculated appearance of the bones simulating a polycystic condition, with thinning and expansion of the cortex. There is no periosteal reaction.

The radiolucent areas usually contain unerupted teeth which may erupt at a later date. Many teeth may be missing and those already erupted are irregularly spaced.

b. Osteogenesis Imperfecta (fragilitas ossium).—There is defective bone formation of the entire skeleton which is prone to multiple and repeated fractures. It is a congenital and hereditary disease and is found from birth to old age.

The patient usually presents blue sclera of the eyes. There are distinct dental abnormalities in this disease with concurrent dentinogenesis imperfecta.

The jaws are thin, with coarse-meshed spongiosa, and the teeth present poorly calcified crowns and fine short roots.

The bones of the cranium are extremely thin.

c. Osteopetrosis (Albers-Schönberg disease, marble bones).—There is a generalized increased activity of the bones of the skeleton. The medulla is obliterated, the cortex thickened, but there is no increase in the size of the bones. Multiple fractures occur. Its onset appears in childhood and the homogeneous X-ray appearance of the bones has suggested the name of marble bones.

The jaws may be so completely sclerosed that the teeth will hardly show in the radiograph.

d. Leontiasis Ossea.—There is extensive periosteal and endosteal proliferation of the bones of the face and cranium. It starts early in life and may be of congenital origin.

The prominent jaws show marked radio-opacity and expansion and there is much hyperplasia of the alveolus.

The teeth do not appear to participate in the excessive bone hyperplasia. There may be retarded eruption and abnormal spacing.

e. Paget's Disease (osteitis deformans).—This disease is characterized by a slowly progressive deformity of some of the bones of the skeleton.

Decalcification and resorption of the bone produce an irregular osteoporosis. The bone becomes softened and bends and loses its shape. The resorbed bone may be replaced by fibrous tissue.

New bone deposition may accompany or follow the loss of bone structure and present a radiographic picture of generalized opacity with a mortar-like granular appearance. This is a disease of late middle life and it is very rare for only a single bone to be affected.

The radiographic changes are distinctive.

Mandible and maxilla: The early changes are confined to open criss-cross trabeculation, areas of various stages of decalcification, and cyst-like formations. There may be a number of scattered, small opaque deposits in the involved area. Later there may be enlargement of the bones, the trabeculation becoming more closely knit, and widespread areas of radio-opaque osteosclerosis.

Skull: It is usual to describe osteolytic and productive phases in the progress of the disease in the skull. These are collateral, but there may be a preponderance of either aspect. The radiograph shows an uneven thickening and overgrowth of the calvarium. The periphery is irregular, and the combination of radiolucent and radio-opaque areas distributed in the bone substance presents a fluffy or cotton-wool appearance. In some cases the bones of the base of the skull appear as massive, dense, ivory structures.

Teeth: The outstanding features are the signs of resorption of the roots of the teeth in the involved area and concurrent hypercementosis.

Long bones and extremities: These are thickened and deformed as a result of the bowing and bending. There are areas of rarefaction and much widening of the shafts of the bone.

Pelvis and spine: The picture is a mixture of the osteolytic and productive reactions.

f. Cleidocranial Dysostosis.—There is a retardation or partial failure of the development of bones ossified in membrane, such as the clavicles and membrane bones of the skull.

It is a congenital and familial condition.

The following are the main radiological appearances:—

Clavicle: Stunted growth, or entirely absent.

Head: Unossified areas, patency of fontanelles, thin walls.

Face: Small and narrow.

Maxilla: Suppressed development and micrognathous.

Mandible: Rarely affected.

Teeth: Increase in odontogenic activity with frequent supernumerary and geminated teeth. The deciduous teeth may be retained longer. The permanent teeth are delayed or inhibited in their eruption and grossly misplaced. The enamel is well formed, but there is much deformity of the roots.

g. Eosinophilic Granuloma.—The condition is identified as a destructive lesion, usually confined to a single bone. The mandible is a favourite site. The radiographic appearance is that of an area of destruction, localized and irregular, with no particular distinctive features. There may be concurrent bone repair. The teeth, if present, appear to be standing without support. This lesion is only identified histologically when mature leucocytes and eosinophilic myelocytes are found in a large granulomatous mass.

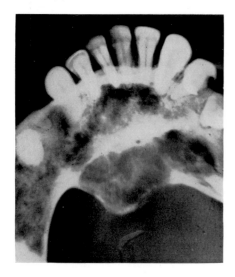

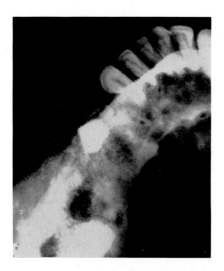

Figs. 776, 777.—Osteitis fibrosa cystica in a female, aged 42 years. High degree of calcification of the mandible with resorption of the bone trabeculation. The picture is that of osteoporosis with pseudocystic areas which are in fact osteoclastomata. The other bones affected were the upper ends of the humerus and femur, pelvis, and bones of the hands and feet.

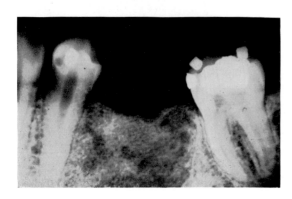

Fig. 778.—Fibrous dysplasia of bone, |56 region, in a female patient, aged 18 years. Localized area of early resorption of the spongiosa, producing the appearance of indefinite rarefaction. The unusual feature is the thinning and expansion of the alveolar marginal bone. Lesion confirmed by microscopic examination after biopsy.

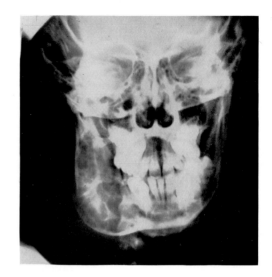

Fig. 779.—Fibrous dysplasia of the right mandible in a female, aged 17 years. The lesion is unilateral, extending from the lower right canine region to the mandibular notch. The appearance is that of a large multilocular cyst with gross expansion of the bone. No other bones involved. Complete absence of teeth on this side of the mandible.

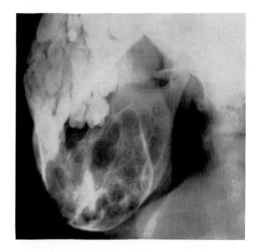

Fig. 780.—Fibrous dysplasia of the left mandible in a female, aged 8 years. The lesion extends from the symphysis menti up the ramus to the region of the lingula of the inferior dental canal. The radiograph shows the characteristic rarefied trabeculated appearance simulating cystic disease, with broadening and expansion of the bone. No teeth are seen in the involved area. This was the only lesion in the skeleton.

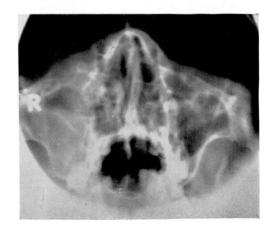

Fig. 781.—Fibrous dysplasia of the right maxilla in a male, aged 26 years. Unilateral involvement of the body of the right maxilla obliterating the maxillary sinus. The condition has spread to the floor of the right orbit, which shows a loss of bone structure and an upward convexity of bone expansion.

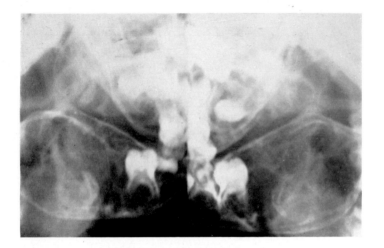

Fig. 782.—Fibrous dysplasia of bone (cherubism). Bilateral involvement of the maxillæ and mandibles giving the patient, a boy aged 8 years, a cherubic appearance. Clinically, both jaws were bulging outwards to form a peculiar rounded swelling of the face.

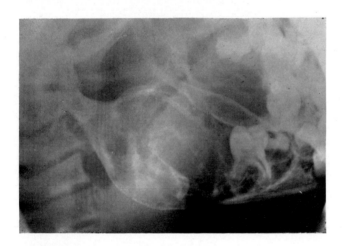

Fig. 783.—Lateral oblique view of the right side of *Fig. 782.* The pseudo-polycystic condition is involving the right mandible from the first molar region to the mandibular notch. The cortex is abnormally thinned, but the bone expansion is laterally, orally, and into the spheno-maxillary fossa. The coronoid process is non-existent. The first lower permanent molar tooth is unerupted and there is no sign of the other two molar teeth.

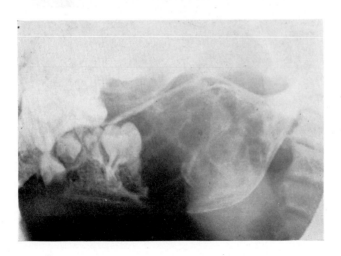

Fig. 784.—Lateral oblique view of the left side of *Fig. 782.* The radiographic appearance is similar to that of the right side of the mandible, but there is no obvious expansion into the mandibular notch. The condylar process is not involved.

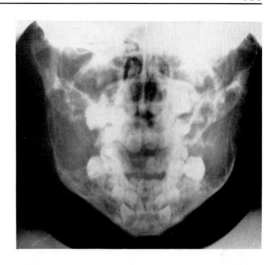

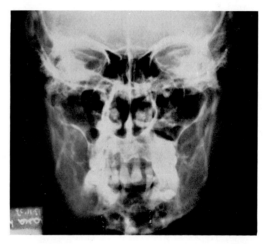

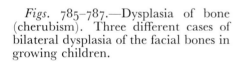

Figs. 785–787.—Dysplasia of bone (cherubism). Three different cases of bilateral dysplasia of the facial bones in growing children.

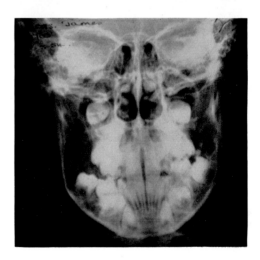

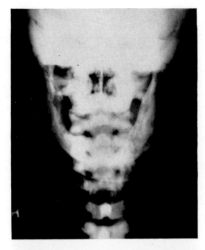

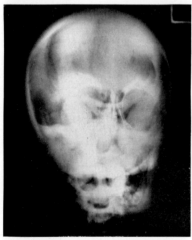

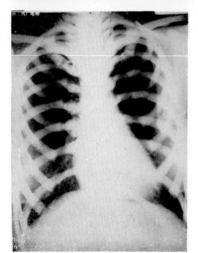

Fig. 788.—Albers-Schönberg disease. Increased density of the facial bones and the frontal bones. Osteopetrosis of the bodies of the upper cervical vertebræ.

Fig. 789.—Albers-Schönberg disease. The postero-anterior view shows that the calvarium is unduly thickened, with widespread areas of opacity.

Fig. 790.—Albers-Schönberg disease. Homogeneous density of all the ribs. Both clavicles are similarly involved.

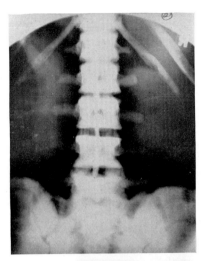

Fig. 791.—Albers-Schönberg disease. Well-developed osteopetrosis of the lumbar vertebræ, the transverse processes, and the sacrum. The innominate bones show bone changes.

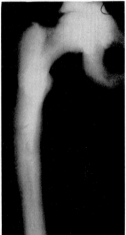

Fig. 792.—Albers-Schönberg disease. The shaft and upper end of the right femur, its neck, and the condylar head all show widespread opacity with obliteration of the medullary cavity of the bones. The hip-joint cavity cannot be seen. There is no actual increase in the size of the bones.

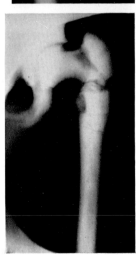

Fig. 793.—Albers-Schönberg disease. The left femur is completely involved by the disease and presents a comminuted fracture in the inter-trochanteric region. The excessive calcification of the bones results in increased brittleness.

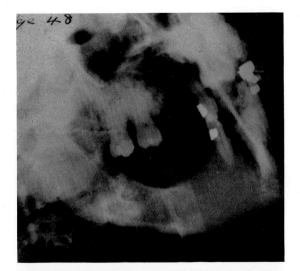

Fig. 794.—Paget's disease in a female, aged 48 years, with painless swelling of the right side of the face of four years' duration. The radiograph shows an irregular opaque mass around the upper right second and third molar teeth.

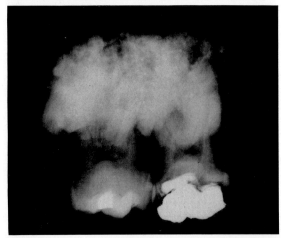

Fig. 795.—Paget's disease. The upper right second and third molar teeth excised, radiographed, and examined histologically. The report was "resorptive changes found in the roots of the two molar teeth with gross hypercementosis".

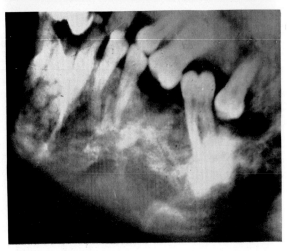

Fig. 796.—Paget's disease. The left mandible presents widespread areas of rarefaction, decalcification, and sclerosis. The lower left third molar is enclosed by a mass of hypercementosis. The mottled appearance is characteristic. There is no irregularity of the lower border of the mandible and no expansion of the bone. The alveolar process is markedly thickened.

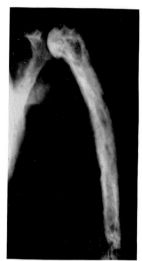

Fig. 797.—Paget's disease. The left humerus presents the typical "moth-eaten" appearance of Paget's disease. The whole of the shaft is involved, with areas of rarefaction interspersed with deposition of new bone formation. The humerus shows the characteristic bowing and bending of the bone. The scapula is also involved.

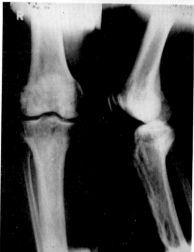

Fig. 798.—Paget's disease. The lower end of the right femur is riddled with multiple small radiolucent areas. The upper third of the right tibia shows loss of the anterior cortical bone, with rarefied spongiosa. There does not appear to be any periosteal new bone formation accompanying the large amount of bone resorption.

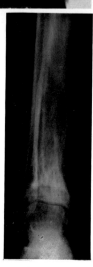

Fig. 799.—The lower end of the right tibia exhibits a cyst-like change, as a result of the bone resorption. The new structure of irregular trabeculation has replaced the old bone formation. There is widening of the shaft in this region, accompanying the osteoporosis, which will eventually show deformity. This depicts the spongy type of the disease.

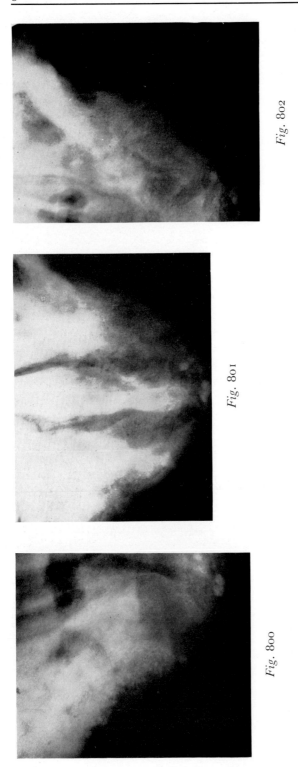

Fig. 802

Fig. 801

Fig. 800

Figs. 800–802.—Paget's disease. Occlusal views of the upper jaw.

Fig. 800.—The midline synchondrosis of the two palatine processes of the maxillae shows dense irregular thickening, extending along its whole length, from before backwards.

Fig. 801.—The incisor, canine, and premolar regions on both sides show a loss of the normal trabeculation, replaced by areas of rarefaction and osteoporosis with a few small isolated areas of opacity.

Fig. 802.—The molar regions exhibit massive deposition of thickened sclerotic opaque bone.

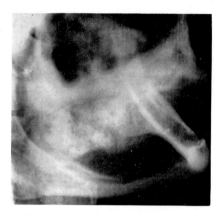

Figs. 803, 804.—Paget's disease. Extra-oral views of the same patient as in Figs. 800–802. Diffuse enlargement of the maxillæ and thickening of the alveolar ridge. The macrognathic changes in this patient are confined to the overgrowth of the cranium and maxillæ. The outstanding feature shown in these views is the almost complete absence of any involvement of the mandible.

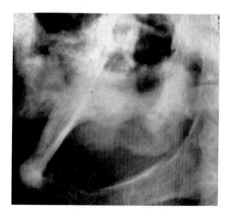

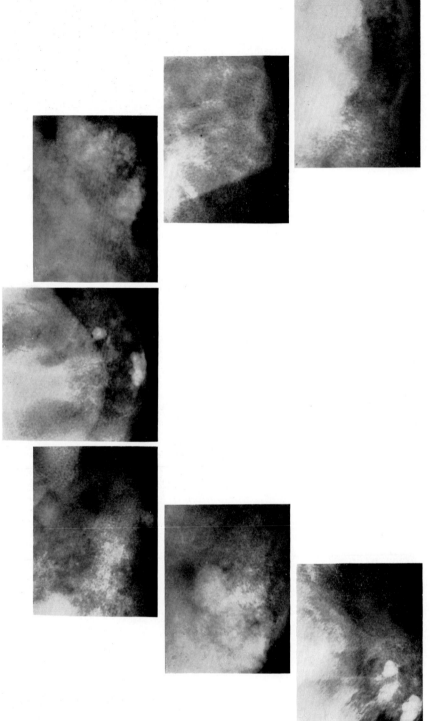

Fig. 805.—Paget's disease. Intra-oral view of the upper jaw. These radiographs present the more commonly recognized features of multiple diffuse areas of osteolytic activity. Normal trabeculation has been replaced by areas of variation in radio-density, some of decalcification and others with irregular patches of opacity, many confluent in formation. The radiographic appearances simulate in many respects chronic diffuse sclerosing osteomyelitis, which is discounted when associated with the history given by the patient of the slow progress of the condition, unassociated with pain.

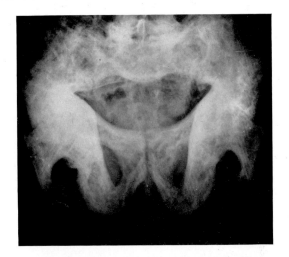

Fig. 806.—Paget's disease. The pelvis presents a mixture of the osteolytic and productive types of the disease. The spongy type shows widening of the bone with criss-cross trabeculation, and in the amorphous type the bone texture is of a homogeneous opacity.

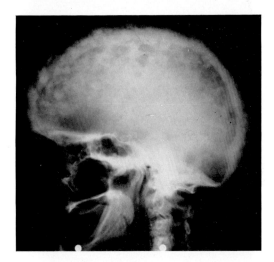

Fig. 807.—The osteolytic skull in Paget's disease. The combination of radiolucent and radio-opaque areas distributed in the bone substance presents a fluffy or cotton-wool appearance. The irregular calcification is clearly depicted, together with the uneven thickening of the outer and inner tables of the skull. The sutures are obliterated.

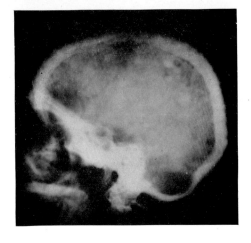

Fig. 808.—The productive skull in Paget's disease. The thickness of the calvaria is greatly increased, and the bones of the base of the skull appear as massive dense ivory structures. There are concurrent osteolytic changes, with islands of dense bone scattered over the bone surface.

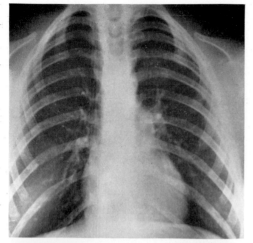

Fig. 809.—Cleidocranial dysostosis. Bilateral absence of the clavicles due to aplasia.

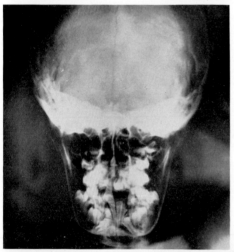

Fig. 810.—Cleidocranial dysostosis. Cranial sutures not completely closed. The maxilla appears to be disproportionately small.

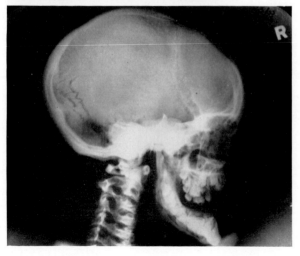

Fig. 811.—Cleidocranial dysostosis. The superior part of the frontal bone shows a large unossified area with no inner or outer tabular walls. The anterior fontanelle is still patent. The maxilla is micrognathous due to retardation or suppression in development. The zygomatic bones and the maxillary sinuses are undeveloped. The mandible is not affected but appears to be prognathous. The mastoid processes are opaque.

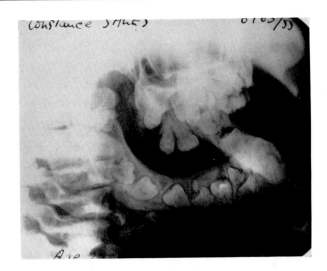

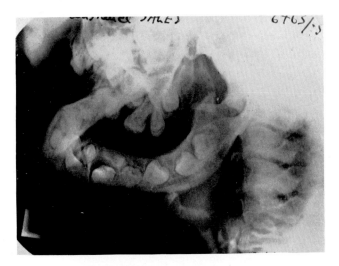

Figs. 812–814.—Cleido-
cranial dysostosis. Right and
left lateral oblique and occlusal
views. Female, aged 22 years.
All the permanent mandibular
teeth appear to be present, but
unerupted. Many show various degrees of version, some
misplaced, and the third molars
are impacted. There are a
number of unerupted supernumerary teeth. The enamel
of the teeth is well formed. The
patient stated that she retained
a number of her deciduous
teeth until the age of 14 years.

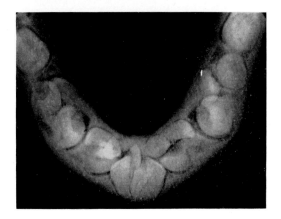

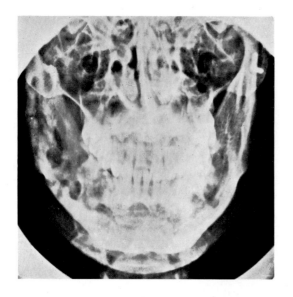

Fig. 815.—Eosinophilic granuloma. Postero-anterior view of the jaws shows multiple, well-defined radiolucent areas distributed throughout the whole expanse of the mandible. The appearance simulates a widespread destructive bone lesion such as chronic osteomyelitis, or even a bilateral bone dysplasia.

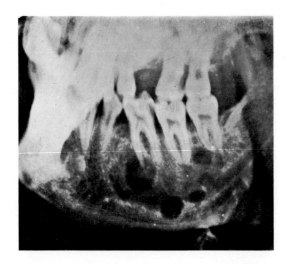

Fig. 816.—Eosinophilic granuloma. Lateral oblique view of the left mandible. There are many cyst-like formations. Although it may appear that some of them are associated with the roots of the molar teeth, there is no connexion with the apices. It is due to an overlapping of the radiolucent shadows of the granuloma on to those of the teeth. The condition could be mistaken for an ameloblastoma.

Index